Clinical Talk

Core Clinical Medicine

CLINICAL TALK

Series Editors: Andrew Goldberg *(University College London and the Royal National Orthopaedic Hospital NHS Trust, Stanmore, UK)*

Gerard Stansby *(University of Newcastle and Freeman Hospital, Newcastle Hospitals NHS Trust, UK)*

Published:

Surgery: Problems and Solutions
Revision Questions in Undergraduate Surgery
edited by Andrew Goldberg (University College London and the Royal National Orthopaedic Hospital NHS Trust, Stanmore, UK) and Gerard Stansby (University of Newcastle and Freeman Hospital, Newcastle Hospitals NHS Trust, UK)

Cardiology to Impress: The Ultimate Guide for Students and Junior Doctors
by Kathie Wong, Edith Ubogagu and Darrel Francis (Imperial College London, UK)

CLINICAL TALK

CORE CLINICAL MEDICINE

Gordon W. Stewart
University College London, UK

Series Editors
Andrew Goldberg
University College London and the Royal National Orthopaedic Hospital NHS Trust, Stanmore, UK
Gerard Stansby
University of Newcastle and Freeman Hospital, Newcastle Hospitals NHS Trust, UK

ICP
Imperial College Press

Published by

Imperial College Press
57 Shelton Street
Covent Garden
London WC2H 9HE

Distributed by

World Scientific Publishing Co. Pte. Ltd.
5 Toh Tuck Link, Singapore 596224
USA office: 27 Warren Street, Suite 401-402, Hackensack, NJ 07601
UK office: 57 Shelton Street, Covent Garden, London WC2H 9HE

British Library Cataloguing-in-Publication Data
A catalogue record for this book is available from the British Library.

Clinical Talk
CORE CLINICAL MEDICINE

ISBN-13 978-1-84816-576-2 (pbk)
ISBN-10 1-84816-576-5 (pbk)

Typeset by Stallion Press
Email: enquiries@stallionpress.com

Printed in Singapore by Mainland Press Pte Ltd.

Contents

INTRODUCTION

The point of this book is to give the first-year-clinical student an overview of clinical medicine. The knowledge base which an incoming student faces is very daunting: the chapters here are an attempt to give a digestible survey of the core problems in each of the main systems of the body, as seen in a British hospital ward.

In some cases we consider the 'failure syndromes' of the body, what happens when (say) the heart fails, giving the well-known syndrome of 'cardiac failure'. Some other systems can be considered in the same way. Although one always tries to diagnose and treat the basic problem, it is often the case in medicine that the underlying diagnosis does not matter, for it is either not known or is ancient history. The damage done by the disease is there; the disease is untreatable or has run its course, and the job of the doctor is to cope with the problems associated with the failing system.

Some system failures (e.g. cardiac, respiratory, liver, renal) follow a simple linear progression. But when other systems fail, things can deteriorate along a number of different paths. For example, 'gut failure' can follow a number of routes. For this kind of problem I have produced 'maps', illustrating in a simple form the common avenues of progression that the patient may follow from perfect health to serious illness.

I have done neurology differently. I have divided it up into 9 'dysfunction syndromes' which are roughly anatomical. Just about a fifth of this book is neurology. No apologies: the brain is so much more complex.

The 20 or so syndromes described here make up about 80% of routine general internal medicine, so understanding of these system failures is a fundamental knowledge base for the practice of medicine. Know this book and know it well. All else is built upon it.

Intersecting with these 'system failure' sections there is a description of the major pathological processes that cause disease. Despite the huge number of different identifiable diseases, the fundamental pathologies that underlie these diseases (infection, cancer etc) number only half a dozen or so.

Chapter 4 looks at clinical medicine in another way: 'Ten Presenting Problems' (a very brief outing into diagnostic medicine), 'Ten Emergencies' (emergencies are obviously vital to know about), 'Ten Tests' (so that you can use them wisely) and 'Ten Drugs' (ditto).

At the end there is a list of abbreviations and what I hope is a comprehensive glossary defining the terms and expressions used in this book and on the wards.

As an incoming clinical student you have a great deal to learn. You have to move forward on a very broad front. You have to develop your clinical skills of history taking and examination; you have to learn how to behave as a doctor within the clinical team and in front of patients; you have to build a 'knowledge base' of human disease (of which this book is really an extended syllabus); you have to understand the tests that are available: how they work, what they tell you and how reliable they are; you have to know the best available treatments.

The single best way to learn is to see as many patients as possible, then to read up on the different aspects of medicine which the cases highlight. This method might be known as 'case lore'. You need to pay attention to pathology so that you can really understand what is going on inside the patient. Get to as many post-mortems you can.

Some students keep a box of cards with a short summary of each disease on it. You can amass about 500 in the course of your time in clinical school, adding new cards and modifying old ones as you see more patients. There is something satisfying about this. 'Here is my knowledge base', the box seems to say.

Remember that your key skill as a doctor remains diagnosis. That is why patients will come to you, as a valued expert.

1

The Pathological Processes

The body can be attacked in a series of ways, which produce the system failures later in this book. The following paragraphs summarise the essential features of these generic kinds of faults, which can affect any system. The treatment of any one patient typically involves a mixture of two regimes, one aimed at the pathological process, the other aimed at the failure of the system which is affected.

It is very important to understand pathology. You will think me terminally sad for admitting this, but I read path books in bed at night (especially those of my former colleague Neville Woolf). They give you insight into what is happening to your patients.

These pathological processes are summarized in Table 1.

1.1. ATHEROSCLEROTIC

We are all subject to a gradual deterioration in the condition of our arteries, which is accelerated by smoking, high blood pressure, diabetes and genetic susceptibility. The walls of the arteries become laden with lipid (in 'plaques'), and later with calcium.

The blood plays its part in this pathology, since its clotting contributes to the clinical dysfunction. Sometimes the arteries are perfect and the thrombosis is entirely the fault of the blood, but most of the time it is the roughened arteries that are the major cause.

Atherosclerotic problems give three kinds of characteristic symptom stories. If the pathology affects an organ whose blood flow changes markedly in response to demand (muscle on exercise, gut digesting food) then there may be a stage in the narrowing process at which the organ has enough blood at rest but not under the increased demand. The patient complains of pain during exercise or, if it is mesenteric ischaemia, blood supply to the gut is compromised and pain comes on after eating. The pain is relieved when the demand for blood flow is reduced. Thus we get the characteristic symptoms of 'angina' (in the heart) and 'intermittent claudication' (legs). The second kind of symptom that can occur is that associated with intermittent arterial blockage caused by small emboli that presumably break up and fail to cause permanent symptoms. These are most evident when they occur in the blood supply to the nervous system ('transient cerebral ischaemic attacks'). Lastly, sudden complete blockage by a major embolus or thrombosis can occur. This corresponds to 'stroke', 'myocardial infarction', 'mesenteric infarct' or 'ischaemic limb'.

On physical examination and investigation, the stroke gives neurological signs consistent with the focal pathology. A myocardial infarct is easiest to diagnose on the ECG. A mesenteric infarct, in which a piece of gut becomes necrotic, causes abdominal pain and always takes the patient into 'very seriously ill' territory: low BP, weak pulse, shock. The ischaemic limb becomes painful and cold, and the peripheral pulses vanish.

Treatment of the failure in the system can be surgical, especially in the lower limbs; by percutaneous catheter intervention in the limbs, heart, sometimes in the renal arteries but rarely in the carotids; or by thrombolytic enzyme, especially for heart and carotid. Preventive treatment aimed at the underlying pathology can be lifestyle and medical treatment for hypertension, diabetes and high cholesterol. Or by never smoking.

1.2. CANCER

Malignant change can happen in any tissue. Lung, breast, oesophagus, stomach, colon, prostate and ovary are the common sites of the localised 'solid' tumours. While the haematological cancers, leukaemias and lymphomas, tend to be spread throughout the marrow and lymphatic system from the outset.

Cancers are randomly occurring things that grow very slowly at first, but which then begin to grow exponentially quickly. As you know, they invade surrounding structures and can spread via lymphatics or the bloodstream ('metastasise') to sites away from the original 'primary' location.

In the solid tumours, the main presenting problems are typically due to the primary tumour, but it is when the metastases occur that the really serious problems begin. Each type of solid tumour has its preferred target destination for metastasis, but there is a lot of variation. When the tumour attains the metastatic stage, it is out of reach of curative surgery, it can have major organ-destroying capability, and it puts increasingly greater demands on metabolic activity.

In cancer there tends to be a gradual accumulation of symptoms. For a long time there is no detectable malignant mass, but the disease relentlessly progresses until it becomes overt in some way.

The treatment of cancer can be as damaging in medical terms as the original disease, taking one into 'immune' and 'haematological' failure syndromes.

There is more about cancer in Section 2.13.

1.3. INFECTION

As organisms, we are very good at repelling invading pathogens, *when healthy*. We live in harmony with many of them, on the skin, in the upper airways and in the gut. It always amazes me how we do not continually suffer pneumonia, always breathing bacteria into our warm wet lungs. The culture of bacteria in the colon is separated from the bloodstream by less than a millimetre of delicate tissue. A biologist will tell you that there are zillions of microorganisms out there in Nature, the vast majority of which would be only too happy to feed on us, and yet only a small fraction have evolved to be true 'pathogens' that routinely cause human disease.

Apart from upper respiratory tract infections which affect us all, and perhaps urinary tract infection in females, the occurrence of infective illness is typically associated with less than perfect health: with sub-optimal nutrition — short on proteins, vitamins and energy; with abnormal anatomy in many forms; and sometimes with frank immunosuppression. Infection is also related to the infecting load of pathogen to which the patient is exposed. Occasionally a clean-living, healthy person is taken over by a catastrophic bacterial infection that just gets lucky and swamps the defences.

Diagnosis of infection can range from the trivial to the very difficult. There may be a large, red, hot swelling, oozing pus on the patient's right cheek; or the patient may have a fever and be shivering with no swelling or pain anywhere. The treatment is often antibiotic-based, but some infections (in which localised bags of pus form) are amenable to surgical intervention.

In the syndrome of severe sepsis (Section 2.11), a massive inflammatory reaction can occur which results in failure of many systems in the body.

1.4. AUTOIMMUNE AND INFLAMMATORY

Autoimmune disease represents a molecular mistake by the immune system, in which the patient's own body becomes the target for immune attack. We cannot do without our immune system, but it has a very hard job to do: it is required to discriminate between self and invader quickly and precisely in order to avoid infection.

The victim of autoimmune disease is more commonly female and of child-bearing age, and this is probably not a coincidence. To the immune system, the foetus is a foreign invader, and the immune system must be modified to avoid it attacking the foetus.

Many organs and tissues can be targeted by autoimmune disease. A whole series of arthritis-type conditions can be seen in the musculoskeletal system. In nephrology, autoimmune attack against blood vessels ('vasculitis') causes renal failure, which often also affects the joints as part of a multi-system attack. In neurology, 'disseminated sclerosis' is the commonest autoimmune disease. In haematology, red cells and platelets can be attacked by 'auto-antibodies'. The 'anti-phospholipid' syndrome is a pro-thrombotic condition in which an antibody to membrane lipids is associated with recurrent thromboses. Autoimmune reactions in the skin are common. In all of these conditions, treatment is aimed at suppressing the immune activity.

The endocrine glands are a very common target (hypothyroidism was the first disease ever to be recognised as 'autoimmune', by Deborah Doniach at the Middlesex Hospital Medical School, sadly now closed). These autoimmune endocrine conditions tend to run their course and end up in destruction of the gland: the doctor's job is to treat the resulting endocrine deficiency. Immunosuppression is not necessary in these cases.

There are other diseases, notably the 'inflammatory bowel diseases', Crohn's and ulcerative colitis, where the clinical disease is due to excessive inflammation. However, that inflammation is not 'autoimmune' in origin, but is a manifestation of a subtle form of immunodeficiency.

1.5. METABOLIC AND ENDOCRINE

The body's biochemistry can go wrong in very many ways. The root cause of the 'metabolic' problem can be genetic, endocrine, renal, hepatic, dietary, intestinal, drug-induced or even psychiatric. But somehow or another, some biochemical abnormality occurs and an organ or function somewhere suffers. I suppose the commonest such metabolic abnormality is atheroma. I am not going to say 'hypercholesterolaemia' here (important though the cholesterol is) because I think that it is more subtle than simple hypercholesterolaemia.

We can include the endocrine diseases under 'metabolic'. Right behind atheroma in the 'metabolic' collection is diabetes (Section 2.6.1), as you know associated with a high blood sugar. In other metabolic disorders, the thyroid can be abnormal, or one of the electrolytes sodium, potassium, acid-base, calcium. High plasma urate is associated with gout. The minerals such as iron, copper and zinc can cause trouble. Lipids are important.

1.6. CONGENITAL

If we include both genetic conditions and acquired conditions that are present at birth, either through environment or accident of development, there must be about 5,000 congenital conditions. No one person can know about them all. It is the paediatricians who are experts here. Many of the inherited conditions are evident in adult medicine, and a very few genetic conditions first show themselves in adult life. Any system can be involved in genetic disease: there is sometimes, but by no means always, a family history; by and large the condition is symmetrical, meaning that it does not favour left over right. The most common in adult practice in the UK? It depends on the geographical locality, but inherited hyperlipidaemias, dominant otosclerosis, cystic fibrosis, thalassaemias and sickle cell anaemia are up there.

It is just now becoming possible to treat some of the recessively inherited disorders by gene therapy, but this is far from routine practice.

1.7. TRAUMATIC

Trauma is the domain of the surgical specialists, especially orthopaedics. Major trauma results in damage to skin and bone and possibly head and spinal column and cord. Haemorrhage is a major problem, and later, infection may complicate trauma.

The internal organs can be affected, especially lung (traumatic pneumothorax), and spleen (which can be ruptured).

Trauma should be obvious as a cause of disease but sometimes the clinical problem can have its onset a long time after the traumatic event, e.g. a spleen rupturing two weeks after a car crash, or epilepsy or pituitary failure developing a year after a head injury.

1.8. DRUG-INDUCED

Lastly we must admit to those diseases that are caused by our own treatment. No drug is perfect. Even penicillin, which can completely cure the patient of a life-threatening infection, can cause severe allergic reactions. Like genetic or metabolic conditions, drug-induced ailments are typically symmetrical in distribution. The liver is a common target of drug-induced disease, but the skin, the gut, kidneys, nervous system, heart and lungs can all be damaged by drug reactions. Some of these reactions are inevitable (neutropenia in chemotherapy), some are truly 'allergic', and some are 'idiosyncratic' toxic reactions. Obviously the key to diagnosis lies in the 'drug history', which will include both prescribed and self-administered medications, and always remembering to ask about known allergies.

Table 1. Pathological Process: Summary.

	Pathology	*Nature*	*Clinical Characteristics*	*Important Tests*	*Treatment*
1	Atherosclerotic	Patchy narrowing of arteries, ± sudden thrombosis.	Pain in some tissues on increased demand; sudden catastrophic event.	Scans of affected organ. Angiograms, Doppler US, ECG.	Surgical or radiologically based intervention with catheters. Thrombolytics.
2	Cancer	Exponential growth of unregulated cellular clone.	Insidious progression. Weight loss, ± abnormal bleeding. Pressure effects.	Scans, especially PET. Biopsy.	Surgery, chemotherapy, radiotherapy.
3	Infective	Pathological growth of unwelcome bacteria, viruses or other invaders.	History covering days. Fever, tachycardia, local symptoms.	White blood count, CRP, scans, cultures.	Antibiotics, ± surgery, fluid support.
4	Autoimmune and inflammatory	Mistaken immune reaction against own tissues.	Younger adult. Relapsing-remitting, painful condition with damage to affected organs.	CRP, autoantibodies ± biopsy.	Immunosuppression.
5	Metabolic, Endocrine	Biochemical damage to target organs.	Often of gradual onset. Symmetrical. Highly variable	Blood biochemistry.	Replacement therapy: endocrine or biochemical.
6	Congenital	Huge variety of problems.	Always symmetrical. Often, a family history.	Scans, biochemistry.	Support the damaged system.
7	Traumatic	Physically damaged tissues.	History usually known. Limbs are major target but by no means always.	X-rays, scans, circulatory assessment.	Surgery to repair if possible. Correct blood loss. Avoid infection.
8	Drug-induced	Toxicity of exogenous chemical.	Hopefully history will be known.	The best test is to withdraw the drug.	Withdraw drug. Support damaged system.

2

The System Failures

In this chapter we will consider the major systems of the body and how they can fail. After the systems, we will look at some important clinical conditions that transcend system boundaries (sepsis, cancer, major haemorrhage).

Typically, for each topic there will be an introductory page, followed by a table and a figure which summarise the main elements of the disease progression associated with failure of that system. Then after the figure there will be some 'Useful Boxes', which illustrate some cogent points.

Some systems are simpler than others. Cardiology is simple; alimentary is intermediate in complexity; neurology is very complex.

The pathological processes that we have just considered attack the various systems to different extents. Atheroma is very important for heart and brain disease. Cancer virtually never affects the heart, but causes many problems in the gut, lungs, haematological and nervous systems. Infection is common in the lungs, skin and urinary system, but is rare in the nervous system. Autoimmunity affects the joints and connective tissue and the brain, and also the endocrine glands.

The *common* diseases that illustrate these interactions are shown in Table 2.0, overleaf.

Table 2.0. Some Intersections in Medicine, showing examples of common diseases in different systems resulting from the various pathological processes. Abbreviations: arthrts, arthritis; HA, haemolytic anaemia; hh, haemorrhage; MS, multiple sclerosis; pyelonep, pyelonephritis; SAH, subarachnoid haemorrhage; sickle, sickle cell anaemia; thal, thalassaemia; tmr, tumour; UTI, urinary tract infection.

	Atheromatous	*Cancer*	*Infection*	*Immune Inflammatory*	*Metabolic Endocrine*	*Congenital*	*Traumatic*	*Drugs*
Cardiovascular	Coronary artery disease	—	Bacterial endocarditis	Vasculitis	Dysrhythmias (Potassium)	Developmental	Tamponade haemorrhages	Many
Respiratory	Pulmonary embolus	Lung cancer	Pneumonia	Fibrosing alveolitis	—	Cystic fibrosis	Pneumothorax	Amiodarone
Alimentary	Mesenteric infarct	Ca of stomach, colon	Gastroenteritis	Crohns, ulcerative colitis	—	Atresia	Ruptured viscus	Steroids
Hepatic	—	Primary, secondary	Viral hepatitis	Primary biliary cirrhosis	Ethanolic cirrhosis	—	Rupture of liver	Very many
Renal	Renal artery stenosis	Renal cell ca	Pyeloneph UTI	Vasculitis	Diabetic nephropathy	Polycystic kidneys	—	Many
Endocrine	—	Thyroid ca	—	Thyroiditis, adrenalitis		Inborn errors	—	Amiodarone thyroid damage
Neurology	Stroke SAH	Secondary, primary tmrs	Meningitis	MS	Diabetic neuropathy	Many	Subdural, extradural hh	Many
Rheumatology	—	—	Septic arthrts	Rheumatoid	Gout	—	(Common)	—
Haematology	—	Leukaemia, lymphoma	Malaria	Auto-immune HA	Deficiencies	Sickle, thal	—	Many

2.1. HEART FAILURE

Cardiac failure (Table 2.1, Figure 2.1) is one of the most common syndromes in the hospital. The likeliest cause is coronary ischaemia, but there are many other causes. The cardiac failure syndrome is characterised by fluid overload, which manifests as peripheral and/or pulmonary oedema. The Frank-Starling curves, which relate ventricular filling with force of contraction (Useful Box 2.1), are important. Fluid overload is the physiological reaction to the defective myocardium.

In only a few cases are we as doctors able to make a substantial improvement in basic heart function. We can repair faulty valves or try to re-vascularise an ischaemic myocardium, but usually one aims simply to manipulate the pathophysiology to relieve dyspnoea and oedema.

You will only very rarely see it, but constriction of the heart due to fluid in the pericardial space, cardiac tamponade, is a possible treatable cause of cardiac failure.

In diagnosis, clinical examination is invaluable: cold clammy skin, medium crepitations in the lungs, possibly the high JVP and ankle oedema. A chest X-ray is vital, serving as it does both to rule out other causes of breathlessness and often positively to diagnose heart failure. The ECG shows you the rhythm and possibly many other features which could point to the cause. The echocardiogram (Useful Box 2.2) can be extremely helpful, but is not always available and is subjective in its interpretation.

Treatment is aimed at reducing the afterload with vasodilators and ACE inhibitors, and reducing the oedema with diuretics. Rhythm control can be very important, especially in atrial fibrillation. Most of these treatments lower the blood pressure, which can reduce renal perfusion pressure in severe cases, which can exacerbate the situation.

Some common cardiological conditions are summarized in Useful Box 2.4.

Table 2.1. Heart Failure: Summary.

Point	*Comment*
Classic features in a severe case	Extreme fatigue. Variable dyspnoea. Oedema, which may be quite gross, and include bilateral pleural effusions, left usually bigger than right. High JVP. Typically in atrial fibrillation. Displaced apex beat, often hard to feel in an older patient. Third heart sound and/or mitral incompetence murmur due to stretching of the base of the valve ('functional' mitral incompetence). Dilated heart on CXR. Possibly patchy shadowing in lung fields (pulmonary oedema). Low ejection fraction on echo. Hyponatraemia on U&E. Loss of muscle bulk generally ('cardiac cachexia').
To look out for	Pericardial effusion and tamponade. Much less commonly missed when echoes are easily available. Aortic stenosis, likewise.
Progression	Typically downhill over many years, with a number of acute episodes requiring hospital admission.
Terminal events	1. Pre-renal renal failure induced by combined action of diuretics and other medications which are hypotensive. 2. Hypoxia secondary to pulmonary oedema. 3. Infection e.g. bronchopneumonia, simply as a complication of the extent of debility associated with an ejection fraction of 10–20%.
Likely causes	Ischaemia, valvular heart disease, hypertension. See Useful Box 2.4.
Rare but treatable causes.	Iron overload, seen in haemochromatosis and some congenital haemolytic anaemias. 'High output' cardiac failure as a result of e.g. thyrotoxicosis, severe anaemia. Bacterial endocarditis which makes valves leaky.
Acute forms	Viral infection, ischaemia.
Tests to be done	CXR, ECG, U&E, BNP (brain natriuretic peptide), echocardiogram, daily weights. Possibly myocardial perfusion scan at nuclear medicine; possibly angiogram.
Treatment (in addition to that of underlying disease)	Oxygen, diuretics, ACE inhibitors; digoxin to control the ventricular rate if necessary (in AF); beta blockers; rhythm control if necessary, including perhaps a pacemaker; low-sodium diet.
Prognosis	Worse than many cancers, please note.

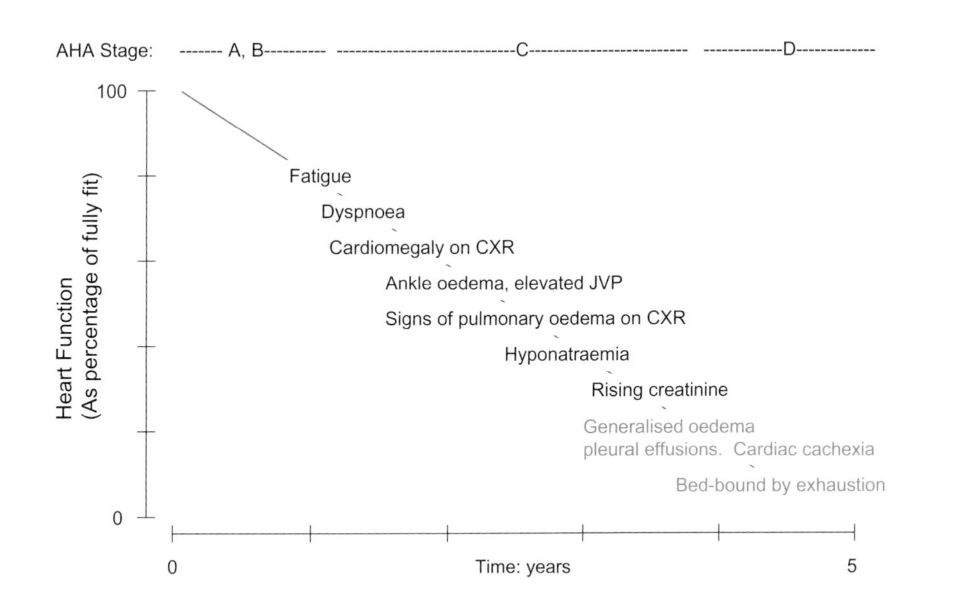

Figure 2.1. The Progression of Heart Failure. The figure shows a five-year time course for a typical patient with ischaemic heart disease leading to severe heart failure. After the cardiac reserve is used up the patient begins to notice fatigue. No obvious diagnosis may be evident at this stage. Later, dyspnoea sets in, then ankle oedema: then a diagnosis can be made. In the terminal stages (green), the oedema becomes unmanageable, the BP drops below 100 mmHg systolic and renal function deteriorates. Abbreviation: AHA, American Heart Association. See Useful Box 2.3.

Useful Box 2.1. Frank-Starling Curves. Named after Otto Frank and UCL physiologist Ernest Starling, the Frank-Starling curves relate filling and ventricular contraction. Basically, the more the ventricle is filled before contraction, the more it pumps out. If the ventricle weakens, it moves to a new curve. To maintain the same output, the filling pressure has to be increased. The body does this by increasing the total amount of fluid in the circulation. The mechanism behind this is unclear, although the answer may lie in the physiological response to haemorrhage. But the end result is fluid overload as the consequence of the body's response to a weakened ventricle. This is how the syndrome of cardiac failure happens.

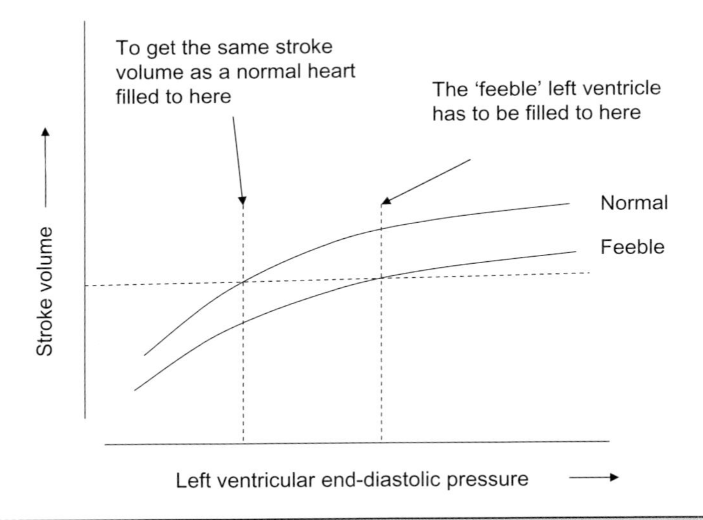

Useful Box 2.2. The Echocardiogram and the Ejection Fraction. There are some very helpful simple tests in cardiology. The ECG is cheap, quick, harmless and very informative. The echocardiogram is a specialized ultrasonic imaging procedure, which follows the movement of the beating heart. It is more expensive than the ECG, is equally safe, but requires an expert operator. Among many pieces of information (function of valves, presence of pericardial fluid), it gives an impression of the ejection fraction, that percentage of the left ventricular volume which is expelled in a contraction. Normally it is about 60%. Those with ejection fractions of 10% are in serious trouble.

Useful Box 2.3. American Heart Association Classification. This is a very useful, practical classification of the severity of heart failure.

Stage	*Description*	*Patient State*	*Treatment*
A	High risk for developing heart failure	Hypertension, diabetes mellitus, CAD, family history of cardiomyopathy	Possibly ACEI
B	Asymptomatic heart failure	Previous MI, LV dysfunction, valvular heart disease	ACEI, beta blocker
C	Symptomatic heart failure	Structural heart disease, dyspnoea and fatigue, impaired exercise tolerance	Above plus possibly digoxin diuretics, aldo antagonists
D	Refractory end-stage heart failure	Marked symptoms at rest despite maximal medical therapy	Above. Possibly palliative care or transplant

Useful Box 2.4. The Common Diseases of the Cardiovascular System.

Ischaemic Heart Disease. Narrowing of the coronaries.

Viral myocarditis. Hardly 'common' but hits young people. Cardiac failure, abnormal ECG.

Inherited Cardiomyopathies. Abnormalities in proteins of muscle contraction. Heart can hypertrophy or dilate.

Rheumatic Valve Disease. This has nothing to do with rheumatoid arthritis. 'Rheumatic fever' is an automimmune feverish disease which follows streptococcal infection. Very, very rare in the UK now, but still happens abroad. The inflammatory process scars the inside of the heart, especially the valves, which become tightened and can leak or become stenosed, or both. Valve problems can present 20 years after the rheumatic fever.

Viral Pericarditis. Common in men in their 30s. Sharp, central chest pain, worse lying flat. ST segment changes on ECG.

Hypertension, meaning high arterial blood pressure, is probably a disease of sodium handling. It leads to thickening of arteriolar walls and patchy unreliable perfusion of organs. Not good for kidneys, heart and brain.

Alcoholic Cardiomyopathy is the weakening of the myocardium caused by the liquid devil.

Cardiac Tamponade is a condition that can result from several causes rather than a unique disease. Presence of abnormal amounts of fluid (blood, inflammatory fluid, malignant effusion) in the pericardial space, preventing the heart from relaxing fully and being filled properly even when patient inspires strongly (creating suction to open the ventricles). Tachycardia, hypotension, high JVP.

Bacterial Endocarditis is infection on the heart valves. The valve webs have no blood supply. Difficult for body to send in defensive war machines (neutrophils) to deal with problem. Valves develop 'vegetations', growing tiny crops of broccoli, which can be seen on echo. Fever, and yet more fever. Embolic sepsis as the vegetations break off and travel around the body.

2.2. LUNG OR RESPIRATORY FAILURE

Easily the most common cause of 'respiratory failure' (Table 2.2, Figure 2.2) is smoking, giving 'chronic obstructive pulmonary disease' ('COPD'): see Useful Box 2.5. The normal fine spongy alveolar structure of the lung is degraded into a coarse, cavitated apology for a lung — 'emphysema'. The lungs are anatomically abnormal and subject to infection, with diminished surface area and gas exchange. Many other pathological processes affect the lung: infection, cancer, fibrosis, trauma with collapse. Or it may be that the lungs are normal but that there is a neurological or muscular problem which weakens the bellows function of the chest.

The patient will complain of shortness of breath. Wheeze and productive cough with purulent sputum are common symptoms. Physical examination will give you an assessment of severity of the respiratory problem: in particular, the degree of dyspnoea. There may be deformity of the chest. Percussion tells you about abnormal dullness and the stethoscope allows you to hear breath sounds (present or absent, vesicular or bronchial, with wheeze and/or crackles).

Hypoxia is picked up by the very simple pulse oximeter and in the arterial blood gases, which give you data on the pCO_2 and the closely-related acid-base status (Section 2.14, 'Blood Gases'). The chest X-ray and then the CT of the chest can be extremely important. 'Lung function tests' involving spirometry can be very useful, indicating 'obstruction' to gas movement, or 'restriction' in lung expansion. The 'carbon monoxide transfer factor' is a very useful number which tells you about gas exchange. Many other tests are possible, but typically the next major test is a bronchoscopy.

Treatment will consist of various combinations of oxygen, bronchodilators, steroids, antibiotics and typically some form of assisted ventilation. Heart-lung transplants are theoretically available but regrettably very rare.

Table 2.2. Respiratory Failure: Summary.

Point	*Comment*
Classic features in a severe case	The patient gives a history of progressive breathlessness on exertion and also at rest in more severe cases, frequently with productive cough. On examination there is evident dyspnoea and possibly central cyanosis. There can be difficulty in speaking in complete sentences. Tests show abnormal oxygen saturations on pulse oximetry. Hypoxia and often hypercapnia with respiratory acidosis are seen on arterial blood gases (see 'Blood Gases, Section 2.14).
To look out for	Pneumothorax. Treatment with the anti-arrhythmic amiodarone (it can cause fibrosis of the lungs).
Progression	Typically gradual, in fits and starts; exacerbations triggered by mild viral or bacterial infections.
Terminal events	Hypoxia, CO_2 retention with respiratory acidosis. Lung infection.
Likely causes of chronic respiratory failure	Smoking: 'chronic obstructive pulmonary disease' (formerly 'chronic bronchitis and emphysema'). Pulmonary fibrosis. Occupational lung disease.
Rare but treatable causes.	Steroid-sensitive fibrotic conditions.
Acute forms	Acute asthma (see Useful Box 2.5). Acute respiratory distress syndrome (ARDS, seen in very sick patients, section 3.5 and Useful Box 2.6). Smoke inhalation. Tension pneumothorax.
Tests to be done	CXR, arterial blood gases (see 'Blood Gases', Section 3.6), spirometry, possibly sputum culture. The chest CT can be very useful. Bronchoscopy when required.
Treatment (in addition to that of underlying disease)	Nebulised bronchodilators; antibiotics; oxygen, often domiciliary. Some form of assisted ventilation. Steroids in some cases, especially severe asthma.
Prognosis	Depends on underlying condition but typically in COPD … 5 years after diagnosis? Maybe longer.

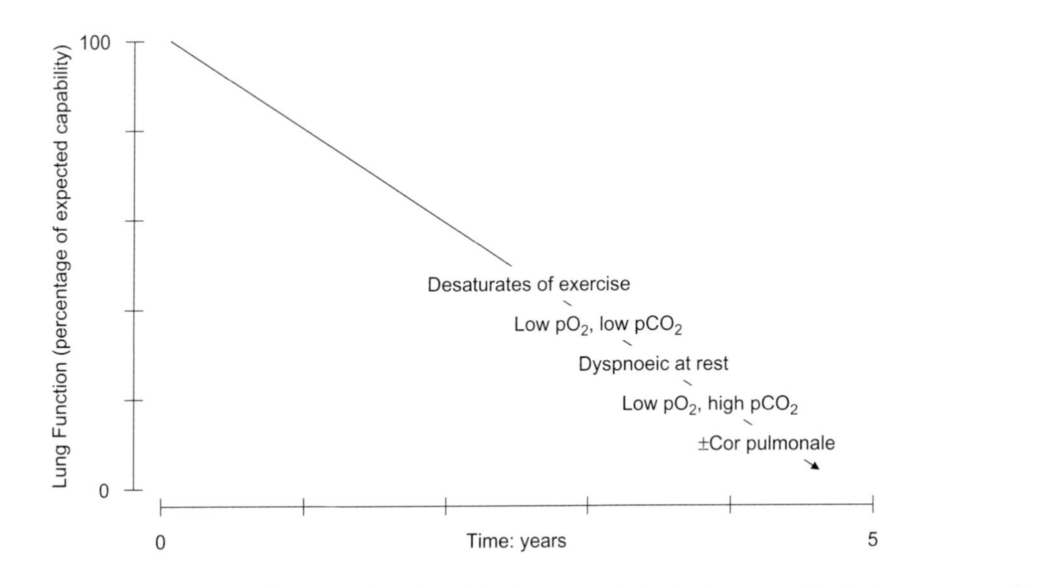

Figure 2.2. The Progression of Respiratory Failure. The function of the lungs is probably best measured by the 'carbon monoxide transfer factor' in respiratory function tests, although this is useful for monitoring. The arterial blood gases and pulse oximetry are used as the standard monitoring measurements.

Useful Box 2.5. 'Asthma' and 'Chronic Obstructive Pulmonary Disease' ('COPD'). Students often find the distinction between these two diseases difficult — 'asthma' is chronic, and there is airways obstruction, so... isn't asthma at least a subset of COPD? No, sorry. Asthma means the intermittently wheezy, immune-mediated, bronchiolar constriction caused by tightening (and possibly relaxing) smooth muscle in the bronchioles. 'COPD', which we used to call 'chronic bronchitis and emphysema', is a condition in which there may be wheeze, but the pathology is different. 'Emphysema' is a state of damaged lung architecture in which the alveoli fuse to form cavities. This pathology can often follow asthma, especially if the patient is a smoker. Although bronchodilator treatment is often given, it is never expected to be as effective as it is in true asthma.

Useful Box 2.6. ARDS: 'Acute Respiratory Distress Syndrome'.

Acute respiratory distress syndrome was first described by American military doctors in Vietnam. Its original colloquial name was 'Da Nang Lung', after the location of the military hospital where it was first recognised. It is a manifestation of widespread inflammatory activity in the lungs, typically triggered by problems outside the lungs, which can be sepsis, haemorrhage, massive blood transfusion or major trauma. The patient's oxygen saturations fall, the CXR shows increasing opacification in both lungs (due to oedema), and the blood gases go bad. Histology shows a widespread inflammatory reaction, with migration of cells and seepage of fluid from the capillaries into the alveoli. Many patients require artificial ventilation.

2.3. INTESTINAL OR GUT FAILURE

Failure of the alimentary system (Table 2.3, Figure 2.3) is not as common a diagnosis as cardiac or respiratory failure but let's consider it. There is failure of absorption of nutrients and fluids, with or without abnormal losses, in the form of diarrhoea. Possible causes include resection by surgery, or coeliac disease, or pancreatic disease, or inflammatory bowel disease (Useful Box 2.8).

The patient will inevitably lose weight, both adipose tissue and muscle. There may be fluid and electrolyte deficiencies. There can be hyponatraemia or hypokalaemia, with or without volume depletion and hypotension. Anaemia is common, possibly iron-, folate- or B_{12}-deficient. The plasma albumin will be low.

One really rare complication of severe malnutrition is Wernicke's encephalopathy: see Useful Box 3.5.

In addition to these generic 'gut failure' problems, the patient is liable to display signs and symptoms specific to the causative disease. Sepsis (often due to *E coli*) and bleeding are common problems in gastroenterology. Cancer is common in the abdomen.

In the investigations, the blood count, electrolytes and liver tests including albumin help in the diagnosis and assess severity. Antigliadin and endomysial antibodies are positive in coeliac disease. It is important to establish if there are problems with the intestinal anatomy, ruling out fistulae and partial obstruction (*complete* obstruction makes the patient very sick, very quickly and typically requires surgical correction).

Treatment involves, if possible, something for the underlying disease. Meanwhile, the immediate problems are treated. Intravenous fluids may be necessary. Nutritional supplements (vitamins, high energy drinks) with or without mineral supplements can be necessary. Parenteral nutrition, in which a lipid suspension is infused into a large vein, is a complex means of treatment, not without risk of infection and liver damage.

Table 2.3. Intestinal Failure: Summary.

Point	*Comment*
Classic features in a severe case	Weight loss; fluid loss; electrolyte and water deficiencies; vitamin deficiencies, resulting in anaemia due to lack of folate and iron. Later, B_{12} deficiency, vitamins D and K.
To look out for	Vitamin/mineral deficiencies other than folate and iron. Malnutrition can be very hard to spot and test for. It's one of those diagnoses that is the sum of a number of impressions: see Useful Box 2.7. Wernicke's encephalopathy can occur. See Useful Box 3.5.
	Weight loss can result from abnormal psychology: anorexia nervosa and depression are two classic causes.
Progression	Depends very strongly on the cause.
Terminal events	Malnutrition: protein and/or calorie and/or vitamin deficiency. Wasting of the body; susceptibility to infection; electrolyte disorders; Fluid depletion which can lead to pre-renal renal failure.
Likely causes	Resection; coeliac disease; inflammatory bowel disease.
Rare but treatable causes.	Lymphoma, perhaps. Don't forget the overactive thyroid in your differential diagnosis here: see Section 2.6.2.
Acute forms	Obstruction, infection.
Tests to be done	Weigh the patient, serially. Blood count, liver function including albumin, U&E, plasma Ca and Mg. Thyroid function. Some kind of imaging (perhaps CT) is always useful. Vitamin levels if possible. B_{12} and folate are routine; vitamin B and others more difficult.
Treatment	High protein foods and drinks. Vitamin (B_{12}, folate, thiamine, A, D, E, K) and mineral (calcium, magnesium, iron, zinc, phosphate) supplements. Some patients require chronic intravenous feeding or fluid support, but IV feeding is inconvenient, toxic to the liver and the indwelling line that is required carries risks of sepsis and/or thrombosis. Blood transfusion may be needed for anaemia.
Prognosis	Very variable.

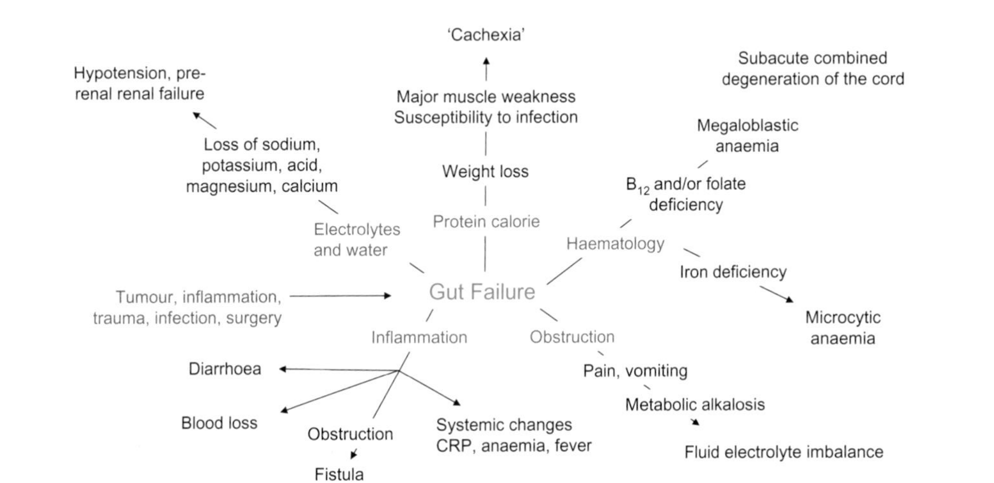

Figure 2.3. The Possible Directions of Pathology in Gut Failure. Gut failure cannot be summarised as a simple linear progression. In the upper half of the map, the three main directions of clinical problems due to deficiencies (fluid+electrolytes; protein+calorie; haematology, embracing vitamins and minerals) are shown. These often go together, but not always. In addition, gut patients often suffer from 'inflammation' (bottom left) in one form or another. This can be as a result of bacterial infection, or the inflammation of 'inflammatory bowel disease': Crohn's or ulcerative colitis.

Useful Box 2.7. The Diagnosis of Malnutrition. 'Malnutrition' is not a simple diagnosis. It is one of those diagnoses that is made from the sum of its parts rather than from one blood test or from one physical sign. There is a great deal of diagnostic exclusion to be done: that the weight loss is not psychological, or dietary in origin; that the anaemia is not due to iron loss or haemolysis; that the low albumin is not due to an inflammatory state (CRP will also be high); that the low plasma calcium is not simply due to the low albumin. Few vitamin deficiencies are easily diagnosable by blood test (B_{12} and folate being the exceptions). The clinical picture can result from many different pathologies. Perhaps one of the most useful points in the diagnosis is the clinical context, that a clear reason why the patient should be malnourished can be identified from the history (short bowel, chronic diarrhoea, vomiting, previous gastric surgery, partial obstruction).

Useful Box 2.8. 'Inflammatory Bowel Disease' is a term encompassing Crohn's disease and ulcerative colitis; two common diseases of young adults characterized by 'granulomatous' inflammation in the wall of the bowel, leading to obstruction, bleeding, diarrhoea, pain, sometimes perforation, malabsorption and 'adhesions' between loops of bowel and other adjacent structures e.g. urinary bladder. The excess inflammation here is likely to represent a 'back-up' or 'reserve' form of inflammation, designed to make up for subtle deficiencies in neutrophil migration.

2.4. LIVER FAILURE

Ethanol can affect many organs (see Section 3.2) but by far its most common victim is the liver. Ethanol is the major cause of liver disease in the UK; let us not forget other causes such as the blood-borne viruses, paracetamol overdose, iron overload, autoimmune damage and the humble gallstone.

The essential features of liver failure are summarised in Table 2.4 and Figure 2.4. The functions of the liver are to metabolise, detoxify, excrete and synthesise chemicals. It transmits blood from portal circulation to the inferior vena cava. Bedside and laboratory assessments focus on measurable parameters which reflect these functions. The patient may be jaundiced, and may show bruising or even frank bleeding. Ascites may occur. When detoxification fails, ammonia levels in the blood rise and the patient becomes drowsy and confused; this state is known as 'hepatic encephalopathy' (Useful Box 2.9).

The blood tests and imaging are vital. The bilirubin, ALT, alkaline phosphatase and albumin are always important, but the prothrombin time is especially prophetic of a gloomy prognosis, signifying decompensation in synthetic function, the liver being the factory for clotting factors.

Defective synthesis can be very temporarily supported by infusion of fresh-frozen plasma, while defective detoxification can be addressed (only incompletely) by the oral administration of non-absorbed antibiotics, to 'sterilise' the gut content, reducing the load of bacterially-produced toxins coming up the portal vein. The ascites can be ameliorated by diuretics, but the major bleeding associated with oesophageal varices is dangerous, requiring transfusion, circulatory support and emergency endoscopy to 'band' the offending bleeder.

It is possible to try and replace the detoxification function of the liver with a machine. 'MARS', the 'molecular adsorbents recirculation system', is helpful but it is expensive and technically demanding.

Table 2.4. Liver Failure: Summary.

Point	*Comment*
Classic features in a severe case	Jaundiced, but not necessarily very deeply. Clinical signs of chronic liver disease should be present if the condition is of long standing. Ascites. Low albumin, prolonged PTT reflecting diminished capacity to make plasma proteins. Hepatic encephalopathy, due to build-up of ammonia, is late and not commonly seen on a general ward.
To look out for	Hypoglycaemia (defective gluconeogenesis).
Progression	Starts with mild derangement of LFTs, which is 'compensated' liver disease: liver dysfunction observable on bloods, but the liver is still doing its job. Later, into 'decompensated', with some discernible loss of function (see Figure 2.4).
Terminal events	GI haemorrhage; infection; encephalopathy; spontaneous and uncontrollable bleeding; aspiration pneumonia.
Likely causes	Ethanol, hepatitis C.
Rare but treatable causes.	Wilson's disease (copper storage disease). Iron overload.
Acute or chronic variants	Acute: paracetamol poisoning, ischaemia due to sustained hypoperfusion and not atheroma. Hepatitis B.
Tests to be done	LFTs; U+E; FBC, including platelet count and WBC; blood glucose; PTT, and other coagulation tests; autoantibodies related to autoimmune liver disease (anti-mitochondrial, anti-smooth muscle); caeruloplasmin for Wilson's disease; iron levels. CXR; ultrasound of liver, possibly CT. Possibly, an ascitic tap (see Useful Box 2.10). Possibly, liver biopsy. Possibly, plasma ammonia if encephalopathy likely. F1s at UCH get the ice for keeping the blood cold on its way to the lab from McDonald's on the other side of the street.
Treatment	Fluids; vitamin K; non-absorbable antibiotics to reduce gut flora. Possibly parenteral glucose to avert hypoglycaemia. Vascular shunting procedures to reduce portal pressure. MARS to detoxify the blood.
Prognosis	In alcoholics, the time from diagnosis to death might be 10 years. In paracetamol poisoning, 3 days.

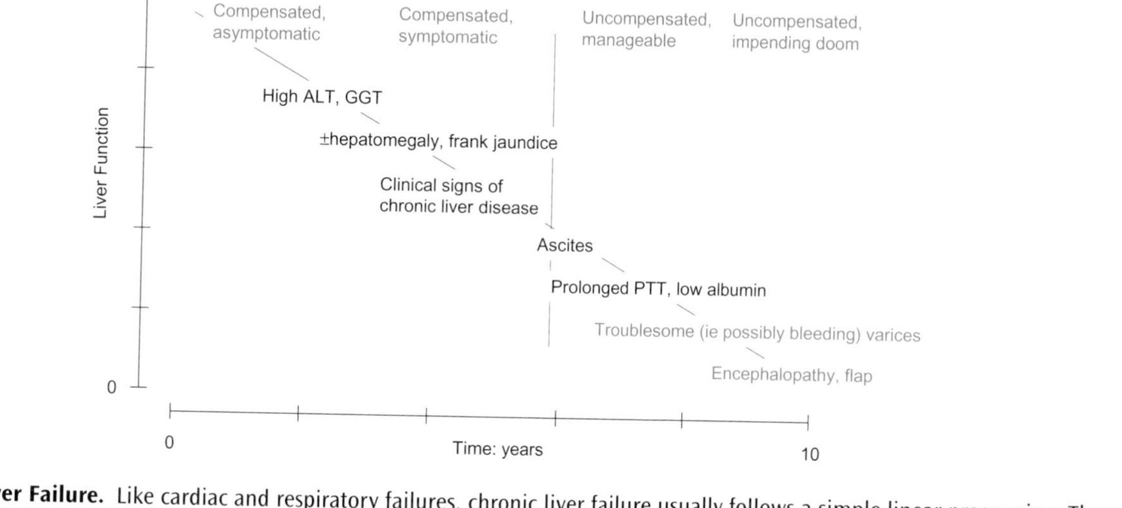

Figure 2.4. Liver Failure. Like cardiac and respiratory failures, chronic liver failure usually follows a simple linear progression. There is an early phase where the abnormality is 'sub-clinical', seen only in the blood tests. Later some physical signs (spider naevi, liver palms, gynaecomastia and testicular atrophy) appear. These early stages are all 'compensated', meaning that the liver is working. The liver disease becomes 'uncompensated', meaning that the liver cannot effectively do its work.

Useful Box 2.9. Hepatic Encephalopathy is another difficult diagnosis, which like that of malnutrition depends as much on the history (in this case, bad liver disease) as on the signs (confusion, drowsiness, even coma). One of the most important circulating toxins is ammonia, which the liver ought to deal with using the urea cycle.

The Table shows the stages of deterioration in hepatic encephalopathy and hyperammonaemia more generally. Don't memorise the numbers: it's the clinical progression implicit in the table that matters. You can imagine that there are many possible causes of this progression.

Stage	*Ammonia: μmol/l*	*Clinical State*
1	<100	Trivial lack of awareness; euphoria or anxiety; shortened attention span; impaired performance of addition (hey, that's me).
2	100–300	Lethargy or apathy; minimal disorientation for time or place; subtle personality change; inappropriate behaviour; impaired performance of subtraction.
3	300–500	Somnolence to semi-stupor, but responsive to verbal stimuli; confusion; gross disorientation.
4	>500	Coma (unresponsive to verbal or noxious stimuli).

Useful Box 2.10: Spontaneous Bacterial Peritonitis.

You will hear about this a lot on the liver ward. A large collection of ascites (perhaps 3 litres) represents a puddle of stagnant fluid that the body has difficulty in policing. The odd bacterium escaping from the gut (which contains billions) can proliferate with minimal hindrance in this ocean of nutrition, free from nasty devouring neutrophils. Thus, often, you will hear the registrar proclaim that he or she has 'done the tap' (taken a sample of the ascitic fluid) and found that the white cell count was 'less than 250', the point being that spontaneous bacterial peritonitis is diagnosed when the neutrophil count in the ascitic fluid is greater than 250×10^9/l.

2.5. RENAL FAILURE

The kidneys are rightly described in clinical medicine as 'the silent system of the body', the point being that as their function falls away there is no loud diagnostic symptom.

Mild renal impairment is often seen on medical and surgical wards, but serious renal failure is rare, certainly compared to cardiac, respiratory or liver failure.

The main measure of renal function is the plasma creatinine. A very important thing to say is that the glomerular filtration rate is an 'inverse' function of the creatinine, an equation of the form $y = 1/x$. This is illustrated in Figure 2.5.

There is a well-defined progression in chronic renal failure (Table 2.5, Figure 2.5). Up to a creatinine of say 150–200 μmol/l (normal, less than about 100), it is asymptomatic. At levels of creatinine above this, the patient becomes increasingly hypertensive, can become anaemic (bottoming out at Hb = 8 g/dl as the creatinine gets to about 350), and then becomes acidotic (with the low plasma bicarbonate of a metabolic acidosis) and hyperkalaemic. Vitamin D metabolism fades and the patient becomes hypocalcaemic.

As the GFR gets down to 30 or 20 ml/min, things get very serious. The creatinine, tripping up and down the steep part of the red curve on Figure 2.5, towards the right, shows much more marked variations from day to day and week to week. Creatinine is not itself toxic but it is a marker for many other non-excreted chemical evils. The three things that are lethal (unless the patient is dialysed) are: potassium ('hyperkalaemia'), acid ('metabolic acidosis') and salt-and-water ('fluid overload': oedema, especially pulmonary oedema with breathlessness).

In acute renal failure (over hours and days), the anaemia and calcium problems are bypassed, but hyperkalaemia, acidosis and volume overload still matter. The urine output takes centre stage as a monitoring measurement.

Table 2.5. Renal Failure: Summary.

Point	*Comment*
Classic features in a severe case	At first renal failure is asymptomatic. Fatigue grows worse as the patient becomes frankly anaemic. Hypocalcaemia due to abnormal vitamin D metabolism becomes evident. In the later stages, there is a pale yellowish discolouration of the skin. In the end-stages, one of three very serious problems will manifest: uncontrollable symptomatic metabolic acidosis; uncontrollable hyperkalaemia (>6.5 mmol/l generally reckoned to be dangerous); or uncontrollable fluid overload, with both peripheral and pulmonary oedema.
To look out for	Obstruction or infection as treatable causes.
Progression	10–15 years. Gradually rising creatinine, with acceleration of rate of rise towards the end.
Terminal events	Without dialysis, the terminal events are either acidosis or fluid overload (with pulmonary oedema) or hyperkalaemia, causing life-threatening dysrhythmia.
Likely causes	Diabetes, ischaemia, chronic infection, hypertension. Glomerular diseases (see Useful Box 2.13).
Rare but treatable causes.	Vasculitis (see Rheumatology section, Useful Box 2.37), multiple myeloma. HIV.
Acute forms	Acute tubular necrosis secondary to hypotension, infection or drugs. See Useful Box 2.12.
Tests to be done	Urinalysis with or without MSU for microscopy (see Useful Box 2.11); U&E; FBC; albumin; US kidneys; plasma Ca and phosphate; blood gases; venous bicarbonate; CXR.
Treatment	In moderate cases it is important to control the BP, commonly using ACE inhibitors which may have a renal protective effect. Vitamin D problems are treated with highly active vitamin D analogues. Subcutaneous erythropoietin for anaemia. Diuretics for fluid overload. In later stages, control acidosis with bicarbonate, high plasma potassium with insulin and glucose. Then it's dialysis and possibly transplantation.
Prognosis	In say a diabetic, gradual deterioration over many years, ending in dialysis. Like liver disease, can move very fast in some patients.

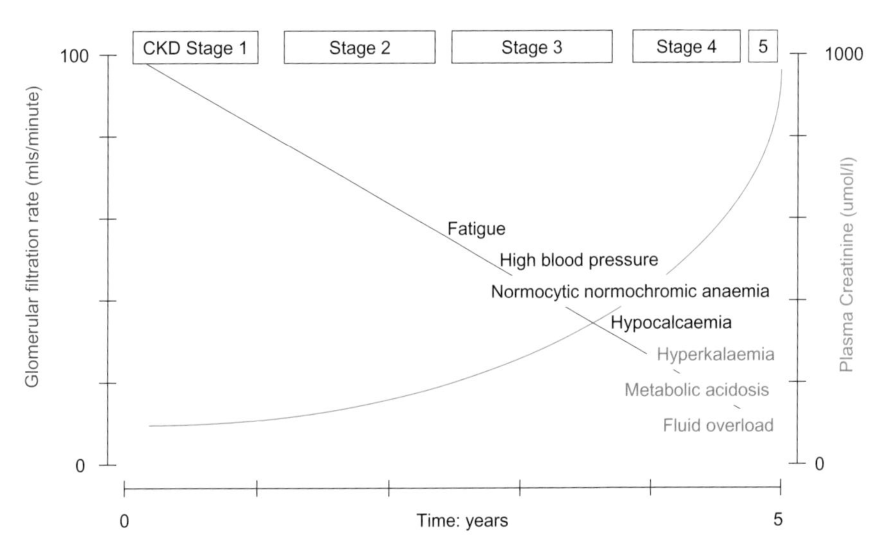

Figure 2.5. Chronic Renal Failure: Progression. The first thing to note is the 'inverse' relationship between the glomerular filtration rate (GFR, in blue, which is the number that really matters here) and the plasma creatinine (in red, which is the one that you can easily measure). As the GFR gradually decreases, the creatinine rises only very slightly. As the creatinine goes from, say, 80 umol/l up to 150, then that corresponds to the loss of 50% of the GFR, which is a lot of GFR. The decreasing GFR is associated with high blood pressure, anaemia, vitamin D deficiency, and then hyperkalaemia, acidosis and fluid overload. The boxes along the top denote the National Kidney Foundation 'stages in chronic renal disease'.

Useful Box 2.11. Urinalysis. Examination of the urine can be very useful for renal diagnosis. There are different levels of sophistication. At the simplest level, the commonly used 'Stix' test strips tell you about presence or absence of glucose, blood, protein, ketones, leukocytes and nitrites (metabolites of bacteria). Examination by microscope (find a microscope!) can show you red cells or neutrophils (both bad news), squamous cells (uninteresting, expected) and 'casts', ejected solid tubular contents made of protein, red cells or white cells. Any cast tells you that glomerular disease is present.

Useful Box 2.12. The Causes of Acute Renal Failure. Diagnosis of the underlying cause in acute renal failure is a major priority. What often strikes me is that the cause is multifactorial, drawn from some kind of combination of factors. Some of these will be immediate: hypovolaemia, drugs (the antibiotic gentamicin is the most notorious), infection (either in the renal tract or elsewhere), myoglobinuria (from mass destruction of muscle: marathon running, trauma, infection, hyperpyrexia), urinary obstruction, or a degree of renal ischaemia; while some will be chronic, and might include diabetes, scarring from previous infection or hypertension or vasculitis.

Useful Box 2.13. 'Nephrotic' and 'Nephritic'. These two words are used to describe two ends of a spectrum of glomerular disease, often, but by no means always, caused by autoimmune pathology. 'Nephrotic' means leaking protein (in grams per day) while preserving renal function, keeping the creatinine low. 'Nephritic' means leaking some protein, often some red cells, and with loss of renal function. Nephrotic patients have acute generalised oedema due to the hypoalbuminaemia; nephritic patients develop renal failure with hypertension and fluid overload.

2.6. ENDOCRINE DYSFUNCTIONS

The concept of a single 'failure pathway' is not useful for understanding diseases of the endocrine system. The individual endocrine glands are certainly subject to failure, often because of autoimmune pathology, but almost as commonly they misbehave by becoming over-active, usually because of a benign adenoma which secretes hormones autonomously.

We are going to consider four endocrine glands: the endocrine pancreas, the thyroid, the adrenal and the pituitary. It is the thyroid and adrenal which can commonly become overactive (the others can too, but it's rare). Pituitary disease is also rare but it is instructive to consider it. We will not consider the parathyroids or ovaries/testes here. Remember that the kidneys can also be considered as 'endocrine glands'. The main miscellaneous endocrine conditions are listed in Useful Box 2.14.

The pathology of the endocrine system is special. Together with the joints, the endocrine glands are a favourite target of auto-immune disease. The endocrine glands are also prone to develop *functional* benign adenomas; these autonomously make the hormone that the original cell type was designed to secrete under proper control. The adrenal, pituitary and parathyroid are especially prone to this. Malignant change does happen in the endocrine glands, especially in the thyroid, but it is much less common than in gut, lung, breast or prostate. Infarction of endocrine glands is rare, but it does occur in the pituitary.

The great beauty of endocrinology as a speciality is that the vast majority of patients can be treated simply and cheaply, by replacing the hormone that is lacking. The treatment may not be perfect. Diabetes mellitus, the result of insulin deficiency, often requires subcutaneous insulin. The dosage is never exactly perfect when compared to the precision of the natural negative feedback loop, but at least you can keep the patient alive for very many years.

Useful Box 2.14. Miscellaneous Endocrinology and Metabolism.

This 'Endocrinology' section is selective. This box is about those topics that we will miss out in the main text.

Calcium. Hypercalcaemia occurs in overactivity of the parathyroid glands ('hyperparathyroidism') and sometimes in cancer, when it can be an emergency. Hypercalcaemia is toxic to the kidneys. There are no very specific symptoms: thirst and polyuria, with abdominal pain, perhaps. Hypocalcaemia, due to loss of parathyroid function or to vitamin D deficiency, causes 'tetany' and hyperexcitable peripheral sensory and motor nerves (also seen in alkalosis and hypomagnesaemia).

Cholesterol. The main thing to know is that about 90% of cholesterol in the circulation is made by the patient. This is why statins, which prevent endogenous synthesis by inhibiting the enzyme HMG CoA reductase, are so effective. 'Low cholesterol diets' are not much good, unless the patient has 'phytosterolaemia' (look it up, it's very interesting).

Urate. Urate is a breakdown product of purines, and therefore of DNA. It is not very soluble and it can precipitate in joints (gout) or kidneys (urate nephropathy). Most cases of hyperuricaemia are genetic in origin, but severe hyperuricaemia can occur in diuretic treatment or in cytotoxic therapy for malignancy. The useful drug to know about is allopurinol, which inhibits conversion of the more-soluble xanthine to urate.

Salt and Water; ADH. Lung cancers are notorious for the autonomous secretion of ADH. This opens water channels in the collecting ducts and the patient reabsorbs too much water, diluting the plasma sodium. The patient can present with a seizure when the sodium drops to about 105 mmol/l.

Hypertension. The cause of 'essential hypertension' remains unclear but I think that it will have a lot to do with some kind of very gradual salt overload. It is certainly true that in those cases where we can define a cause, genetic or acquired, it is often to do with salt metabolism. A classic example is Conn's syndrome, due to hypersecretion of the mineralocorticoid aldosterone.

2.6.1. The Adult Diabetic Patient

The commonest glandular dysfunction is failure of the endocrine pancreas, giving diabetes type one or two (Table 2.6.1, Figure 2.6). Type one typically occurs in younger patients, is auto-immune in origin, and is associated with complete absence of insulin. There is an absolute requirement for treatment with insulin. Without it, ketoacidosis will occur. Type two is commoner and its prevalence is rising rapidly. It occurs in more senior patients, is associated with obesity, a family history, and often with Asian ethnicity. The onset of type two is gradual and the shortage of insulin is not absolute. It can usually be treated with diet and oral hypoglycaemic agents. It does not progress to ketoacidosis but can progress to severe hyperglycaemia, with major osmotic problems.

The long term complications of diabetes are probably due to cellular poisoning by chronically high glucose levels. See Useful Box 2.15.

The kidneys are often a problem. In the early stages, the glomerulus leaks protein but continues to filter. Later, function is lost and gradually the glomerular filtration rate drops, and the patient falls into renal failure. The severity of renal pathology is mirrored by the severity of retinal pathology. Often, neuropathy combined with vascular insufficiency, especially in the feet, are the overt problems for the patient. The rate of progression of 'standard' large-vessel atheroma is accelerated.

The diagnosis is usually made via the blood glucose. The HbA1C is a help; an oral glucose tolerance test is sometimes used in a borderline case.

Treatment of type one diabetes is always with insulin and a suitable diet. Type two is treated with diet, oral hypoglycaemic agents and if these measures do not work, insulin. In all cases intensive education of the patient is required.

Table 2.6.1. Diabetes: Summary.

Point	*Comment*
Classic features in a severe case	Acute: Tendency to thirst and polyuria; weight loss. Chronic: vascular insufficiency, especially in the feet, but also coronaries and carotids. Gradually progressive renal failure, typically closely matched by the diabetic retinopathy in the eyes. Peripheral neuropathy. Lingering infections of feet with breakdown of the skin, possibly extending to osteomyelitis (infection of bone) and gangrene (death of tissue). Ischaemic cardiac problems with abnormal ECGs, acute coronary syndromes, and heart failure.
To look out for	The retinopathy. You won't forget the BP and the creatinine either, will you?
Progression	Gradual — over years.
Terminal events	Renal failure. Heart failure. Infection. Ischaemia (stroke, MI, gut infarction, gangrene of a limb).
Likely causes	Type two — Obesity. Ethnicity. Family history.
Rare but treatable causes	Cushing's disease, acromegaly. Remember the iatrogenic cause: glucocorticoid treatment (prednisolone, dexamethasone).
Acute forms	In type one: diabetic ketoacidosis, In type two: hyperosmolar non-ketotic coma (HONK) occurs.
Tests to be done	Blood pressure. Ankle reflexes. Vibration sense. Fundoscopy Urinalysis especially for proteinuria. Blood glucose, HbA1C, U&E. ECG. Exercise test, echo for heart. Arterial studies if necessary. Blood gases in acute type one cases where DKA is suspected.
Treatment	Insulin or oral hypoglycaemic agents. Fluids if needs be. Monitor doses and blood tests. Specialised nurse practitioners are invaluable in the management of these patients.
Prognosis	Reasonable. Renal failure and blindness are no fun. It is arterial problems that are commonly the terminal events.

Useful Box 2.15. Diabetes Attacks Cells Which Do Not Require Insulin.
The cells that *do not* depend on insulin for glucose entry are vulnerable because the high blood glucose has free access to the interior of these cells, soaking their proteins in toxic glucose. The main targets are nerve and vascular endothelial cells, including the glomerular tuft. Glucose has free entry to red cells: the extent of glycosylation of haemoglobin is used as a measure of diabetic control — the 'HbA1C'.

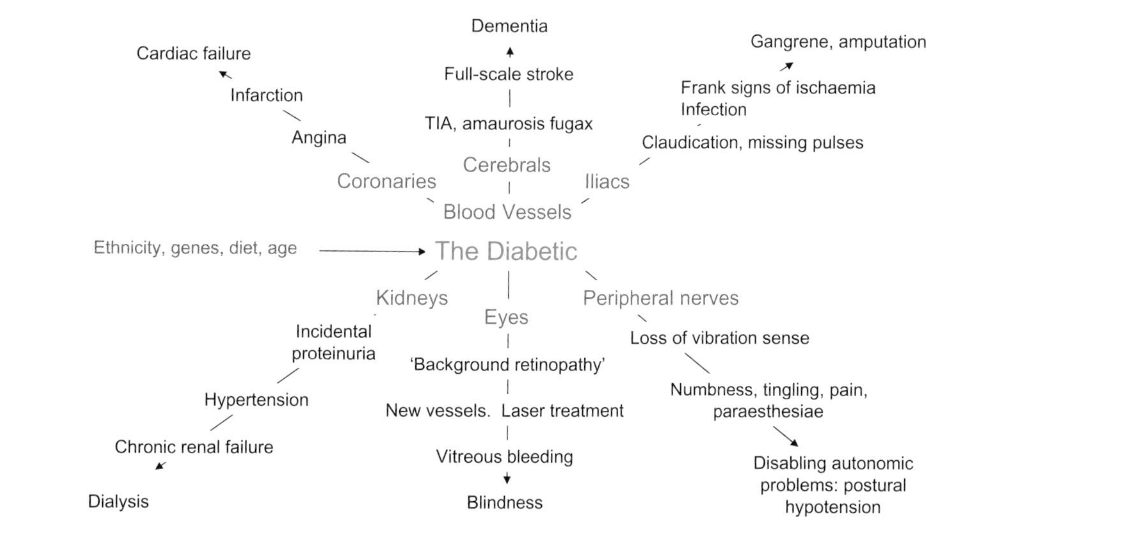

Figure 2.6. Map: The Diabetic. Diabetes progresses very slowly, typically over decades. The six arms of this diagram summarise the main ways in which the patient can suffer. The top three are all related to larger blood vessels. The lower three (kidney, eyes, peripheral nerves) are more 'microvascular' in pathology. By and large they progress together. Perhaps in younger patients the 'Blood Vessel' problems in the upper half of the diagram are slower than in older patients.

2.6.2. Thyroid Dysfunction

After diabetes, thyroid problems are the commonest endocrine diseases. We will consider both hypothyroidism and hyperthyroidism (Table 2.6.2). They are polar opposites in pathophysiology and some of the symptoms and signs are exact opposites (constipation vs diarrhoea, bradycardia vs tachycardia, weight gain vs weight loss) but it is not all so simple.

In **hypothyroidism**, the patient is typically more senior. He or she can present with 'fatigue', that least specific of symptoms. The classical specific symptoms and signs (cold intolerance, weight gain, constipation, dry skin, slow-relaxing deep-tendon reflexes) are certainly useful to know about and to look for, but are not often seen.

Treatment of hypothyroidism is very simple. It is traditional to start with a lowish dose of thyroxine to give the body time to get used to the relatively sudden increase in metabolic demand occasioned by increased thyroxine levels.

In **hyperthyroidism** the metabolic rate is stepped up. The patient typically loses weight, has a tachycardia and a tremor. There can be diarrhoea and intolerance of warm temperatures. In the classic autoimmune form known as Grave's disease there is exophthalmos caused by swelling of the extraocular muscles. In more senior patients hyperthyroidism can manifest as heart failure with breathlessness and ankle swelling. Very severe hyperthyroidism can be life-threatening (Useful Box 2.16)

The treatment of an over-active thyroid is typically with carbimazole, which suppresses thyroid function. Beta blockers, usually propranolol, are used to suppress tachycardia and tremor but do not affect the thyroxine level itself. Later, something radical can be done about the thyroid, usually treatment with radioactive iodine (which is concentrated in the thyroid), but sometimes patients have surgery (a 'sub-total thyroidectomy').

Table 2.6.2. Thyroid Dysfunction.

Point	*HYPOTHYROID*	*HYPERTHYROID*
Classic features in a severe case	A very slowly progressive deterioration in an older patient. Fatigue, hoarse voice, constipation, hypothermia, coldness, dry skin, hyponatraemia, macrocytosis, bradycardia, slowly-relaxing tendon reflexes. Hypercholesterolaemia.	A younger patient, 20–55. Weight loss, tremor, difficulty with warm temperatures, anxiety, maybe exophthalmos. Tachycardia, sometimes AF, goitre, possibly with a bruit. In older patients, 'high-output' cardiac failure.
To look out for	Hypopituitarism: TSH will be low, not high.	Drying of the corneas in severe exophthalmos.
Progression	Very gradual.	Over months.
Terminal events	Hey, none of these please.	'Thyroid storm' with cardiac failure and arrest can happen.
Likely causes	Autoimmune thyroiditis; previous treatment with radioactive iodine, or surgery.	Autoimmune most often.
Rare but treatable causes	Amiodarone, hypopituitarism.	Amiodarone (again).
Acute forms	Thyroiditis.	'Thyroid storm' (Useful Box 2.16).
Tests to be done	T4 (low, obviously), TSH (very high in a typical case).	T4 (high), TSH (undetectable).
Treatment	Thyroxine: start it slowly. Final dose will be between 100 and 150 μg/day.	Carbimazole plus beta blocker; perhaps radio-active iodine or thyroid surgery.
Prognosis	Excellent.	Excellent.

Useful Box 2.16. Thyroid Storm. This is a very unusual thing, but if the thyroid goes completely berserk, then extreme thyrotoxicosis becomes life-threatening. There is fever and tachycardia so fast that the ventricles become mechanically inefficient, giving heart failure. There is marked tremor, anxiety and confusion. It can happen after thyroid surgery, if the patient has not been properly 'prepared' (that is, chemically suppressed) beforehand.

2.6.3. Adrenal Dysfunction

In adrenal disease, autoimmune pathology and sometimes tumours, or infections like HIV/AIDS or TB can cause destruction of the glands. The under-and overactive conditions are compared in Table 2.6.3. and The clinical picture of **adrenal failure** is a mixture of mineralocorticoid deficiency (a sodium and water-losing state with hypovolaemia, hypotension, hyponatraemia and hyperkalaemia) and glucocorticoid deficiency (hypoglycaemia when starved). 'Addison's disease' (=adrenal failure) is rare but it's in here because it is difficult to diagnose, easy to treat, and fatal if left untreated. It presents with very chronic fatigue. The classic signs are hypotension with pigmentation of the skin. There can be patchy pigmentation of the mucosal surfaces inside the mouth. The blood tests show a low plasma sodium, high potassium, a mild metabolic acidosis, and possibly a degree of (pre-renal) renal impairment.

The definitive diagnostic test is a 'short synacthen test', in which a dose of synthetic ACTH is given after a basal plasma cortisol is taken. Two further plasma cortisols, at 30 and 60 minutes, are then taken, and the cortisol should rise above 550 nmol/l at some point if the adrenal glands are functioning.

Adrenal over-activity is selective between mineralo- and glucocorticoid disorders. It can be due to adenomas of the gland itself, making aldosterone (the hypertensive, hypokalaemic Conn's syndrome, not considered here) or cortisol, giving Cushing's syndrome in which the patient shows central obesity, often with diabetes, hypertension and wasting of skin, connective tissue and muscle. Cushing's syndrome can also be caused by a pituitary adenoma secreting ACTH, or of course by high doses of steroid-type drug medication, e.g. prednisolone.

The diagnosis of either adrenal or pituitary Cushing's is not easy. It involves repeated timed blood samples ('diurnal cortisols'), 24-hour urine collections and MRI scanning of the adrenals. The vexed question of who to test is considered in Useful Box 2.17.

Table 2.6.3. Adrenal Dysfunction.

Point	*UNDERACTIVE ('Addison's')*	*OVERACTIVE ('Cushing's')*
Classic features in a severe case	Wasting disease with pigmentation of the skin. Salt- and water-losing: hyponatraemia, hyperkalaemia, low BP. Tendency to hypoglycaemia.	Central obesity, atrophy of skin ('striae') and muscle ('proximal myopathy'), type two diabetes, hypertension, susceptibility to infection.
To look out for	TB or tumour in the adrenals. HIV/AIDS.	Illicit or unknowing steroid use by the patient.
Progression	Very slow.	Also slow.
Terminal events	Hyperkalaemic cardiac arrest. Hypoglycaemic brain damage.	Many possible terminal outcomes, secondary to diabetes or hypertension or infection.
Likely causes	Autoimmune; withdrawal of previous steroid therapy.	Pituitary or adrenal adenoma. Steroid treatment.
Rare but treatable causes	TB, HIV/AIDS.	Adrenal cancer. ACTH-secreting cancers e.g. lung.
Acute forms	Withdrawal of chronic steroid treatment.	Drug-induced. Malignant adrenal tumour.
Tests to be done	U&E. Short synacthen. Autoantibodies, CT or MRI of adrenals, HIV serology.	24-hour urines for steroids. Diurnal plasma cortisol. 'Dexamethasone suppression test'. MRI imaging of pituitary and adrenals is very useful.
Treatment	Hydrocortisone, sometimes with fludrocortisone.	Metyrapone. Surgery. Treatment for diabetes and hypertension.
Prognosis	Excellent if diagnosed. Dire if not.	Reasonable: but depends on the comorbidities.

Useful Box 2.17. Who to Screen for Cushings? There are a lot of overweight diabetic hypertensive patients out there. Diagnosis of Cushing's is time-consuming. They cannot all be tested. Selection depends on your clinical assessment. The distribution of the body fat is key; the impressive, almost globular, abdomen and moon-shaped face with it's ruddy skin colour, compared with the skinny arms and legs; the quite aggressive blood pressure; the striae on the skin; and the diabetes.

2.6.4. Pituitary Failure

Pituitary failure (Table 2.6.4) is very uncommon, but like Addison's it is vital to recognise it. It can be caused by a gradually enlarging adenoma, or by trauma (which interestingly may have been far in the past), or by infarction. The patient presents with fatigue. There is a typical succession in loss of pituitary function as the gland fails. First to go is LH-FSH secretion, giving secondary amenorrhoea in females and loss of sexual function in the male. TSH secretion fails next, giving hypothyroidism with a *low* TSH. Next it's growth hormone, but this is asymptomatic in adults. ACTH secretion is usually preserved until last, but when it fails, the patient gradually loses glucocorticoid and then mineralocorticoid function.

Definitive diagnosis requires a sophisticated 'dynamic test'. The pituitary-adrenal axis is 'stressed' by the induction of hypoglycaemia by IV insulin. Once the blood sugar has fallen below 2.2 mmol/l, glucose is given. The patient must not be left unsupervised. TRH and LHRH are given at the same time as the insulin. Over a 2 hour period repeated blood samples are taken for cortisol, TSH, GH, ACTH, LH, FSH, T4, and you can see if the pituitary is capable of responding to your three stimuli. Although this is time-consuming and complex, it is a very vital test for your patient; it tells you whether the patient does or does not need a lifetime of hormone replacement.

The presence of a pituitary adenoma has implications for the optic chiasma. See Useful Boxes 2.18 and 2.19.

ADH secretion is *not* usually lost at all unless there is hypothalamic damage: see Useful Box 2.20. Lack of ADH gives diabetes *insipidus*. Typically, such patients are thirsty but the thirst drive will make them drink enough to keep up with losses. It is when they are deprived of water (e.g. fasting for surgery) that they lose water and become hypernatraemic, while excreting an unexpectedly dilute urine.

Table 2.6.4. Pituitary Failure.

Point	*Comment*
Classic features in a severe case	Not an easy diagnosis. Fatigue with some weight loss. Secondary amenorrhoea but this has many other causes. Loss of libido and loss of secondary sexual characteristics: hard to be sure in a mild case and can be misdiagnosed easily as depression or chronic fatigue syndrome. Hypothyroidism may or may not be clinically detectable. Adrenal failure is late. Blood tests can show hyponatraemia and/or macrocytosis. A low T4 with low TSH can mean simply 'sick euthyroid' but it adds to the picture.
To look out for	Presence of an expanding pituitary lesion: bitemporal hemianopia. Adrenal failure: hypoglycaemia.
Progression	Can be very slow, over years.
Terminal events	Hypotension, hypoglycaemia, adrenal crisis.
Likely causes	Prolactinoma. 'Empty sella': presumed previous infarction. Previous head injury.
Rare but treatable causes	Hypopituitarism is easily treated by hormone replacement, but the underlying pituitary disease is harder to treat.
Acute forms	Pituitary apoplexy. The pituitary has a tenuous portal blood supply and is susceptible to infarction, especially in pregnancy.
Tests to be done	FBC, U&E. T4, TSH. Cortisol, ACTH. LH, FSH, testosterone. Then: triple bolus test. MRI scan.
Treatment	Replacement hormones: hydrocortisone, thyroxine, sex hormones, GH for children.
Prognosis	Excellent if you diagnose it. Bleak if you do not, like Addison's.

Useful Box 2.18. Visual Field Testing. As you know the pituitary lies in a bony recess just under the optic chiasma, the junction box for the optic nerves. If there is an enlarging mass in the fossa, its only escape route from the bony cavern is vertically up, pressing on the chiasma. This pressure typically presses on the fibres in the centre of the chiasma: those that are crossing over. Pressure on these fibres leads to visual field problems affecting the temporal fields of the eyes. The irregular shape of the enlarging pituitary makes for irregular field loss in the eyes. Perhaps only one eye will be affected; even then, only a small part of one quadrant of the field. Your technique has to be skilled and robust.

Useful Box 2.19. David and Goliath. Here's something. It has been suggested that Goliath suffered from growth hormone excess, which began before his epiphyses fused, allowing him to grow to a great height (gigantism). The adenoma responsible for the growth hormone pressed up on his chiasma, giving him a bitemporal hemianopia. The nimble David was therefore able to creep up on him from the side and get close enough to smite him down. It does make clinical sense, you have to admit.

Useful Box 2.20. The Posterior Pituitary and ADH. In pituitary disease, ADH secretion is *not* usually lost unless there is hypothalamic damage: the anatomy of ADH-secreting cells is different from other pituitary cells. The bodies of ADH-secreting cells are located in the hypothalamus, and the secretion is made by a neuron-like extension into the pituitary. If the pituitary is harmed, the ADH-secreting cells simply secrete from a new, more proximal, nerve ending.

2.7. NEUROLOGY

Sections 2.7.2.1–9 are about neurology. We are first going to consider the manner in which the pathological processes apply to diseases of the nervous system. Then we are going to look at a way of trying to classify neurological disease, which depends largely on the region of the nervous system which is affected.

2.7.1. Pathological Processes in Neurology

Chapter 1 described the important pathological processes in medicine in general. Here is that list again (Table 2.7.1), as it applies to neurology. These pathological processes in neurology will intersect with the anatomical syndromes in the forthcoming Sections 2.7.2.1–9.

The clinical medicine of neurology is influenced by the special cellular nature of neurons, which are very large, highly sophisticated cells that are very difficult to renew. If the axon is cut it can theoretically re-grow, or if compressed can be rebuilt, but if the cell body dies, then by and large, that's it. Neurones are exquisitely sensitive to hypoxia: 'hypoxic brain damage' is a classic outcome of cardiac arrest or a lengthy difficult birth, and 'stroke' caused by localised arterial insufficiency is the commonest form of neurological disease; even very short periods of arterial obstruction or any form of hypoxia cause major symptoms and disability.

The stringent, picky metabolism of neurones makes them very susceptible to disturbances in other metabolic conditions apart from hypoxia, such as low blood sugar, high blood ammonia, and countless poisons including opiates and amphetamines.

By and large, brain cells are turned over very slowly. Primary brain tumours are therefore rare but do occur sometimes. Secondary metastatic tumours from lung or bowel are commoner. Because they are not turned over, neurones are particularly subject to processes of very slow cellular degeneration, in which insoluble proteins very slowly accumulate in the cell (so-called 'proteinopathies'). Many of these processes are genetic in origin. These disorders give a clinical picture of very slowly advancing, disabling, symmetrical disease without remission, and without much useful treatment on offer at present. The patients require 'support' in all its forms. Alzheimer's and Parkinson's work this way. Creutzfeldt-Jakob disease is an acquired form.

Tumours (and some other 'mechanical' abnormalities) can cause raised intracranial pressure, a very specific neurological problem that we will come to later (Section 2.7.2.8).

The brain is susceptible to autoimmune disease, mainly in the form of 'multiple sclerosis', a remitting and relapsing condition of the central nervous system which is one of the classics of neurology.

The conceptually difficult technique of magnetic resonance imaging is important in neurology. See Useful Box 2.21.

Epilepsy

This is a pathological state that is almost unique to the nervous system (cardiac ventricular and atrial fibrillations are its only equivalent in another system). It is a state of uncontrolled electrical hyperactivity which causes loss of coordinated function. There is usually a focus at which the uncontrolled firing starts, from where it spreads to take over the whole brain. In its classical 'grand mal' form, typically there is loss of consciousness with very obvious uncontrolled muscular contractions. The event is terminated by hypoxia. I suppose that epilepsy is always 'caused by' some underlying pathology, but it can be impossible to define the real source. Known causatives include hypoglycaemia, high body temperature, low plasma sodium, brain infection, tumour, hypoxia, or trauma. Any pathological process that causes epilepsy must always do so by somehow affecting the grey matter. Epilepsy is typically treated with drugs that somehow or another inhibit action potentials.

Table 2.7.1. Summary of Pathological Processes in Neurology.

Process	*Characteristics*	*Classic Disease Example*
Vascular	Sudden onset, gradual recovery of unpredictable extent. Two big vascular problems occur in neurology: the 'stroke' or 'cerebrovascular accident', related to atheroma in the carotids or vertebrals; and 'subarachnoid haemorrhage', a bleed from a congenital aneurysm in the circle of Willis.	Stroke SAH
Infection	Onset over days or hours, or longer in TB. Fever. CRP need not be high.	Meningitis
Metabolic	Unpredictable but symmetrical problems. One or more of: confusion, impaired conscious level, muscular weakness, peripheral neuropathy, fits.	Hypoglycaemia
Tumour	Gradual onset over weeks or months. Asymmetric 'focal' neurology. Possibility of raised intracranial pressure (headache, nausea, papilloedema).	Metastases from e.g. lung
Inflammatory	Onset of an acute attack is over days. Relapsing, recurrent course. In the peripheral nerves, 'Guillain–Barré' is an autoimmune disease affecting motor nerves.	Multiple sclerosis, Guillain–Barré syndrome
Genetic	Always symmetrical. All parts of nervous system can be affected. Although most forms are present at birth, some very slowly-progressive conditions can present in adulthood. Thousands of different diseases.	Huntington's, Charcot-Marie-Tooth
Traumatic	Even if there is no skull fracture, trauma to the skull can damage the brain by causing haemorrhage within the skull (arterial 'extra-dural' or venous 'sub-dural' haemorrhage) or by bruising, known as 'contusion'.	Subdural haematoma
Drug-induced	Symmetrical; confusion, diminished conscious level, fits. History of exposure.	Ethanol, amiodarone

Useful Box 2.21. Magnetic Resonance Imaging

Magnetic resonance imaging (MRI) is vital in neurology but very few medics understand it. Here goes.

The elementary particles in atoms (protons, neutrons, electrons) have 'spin'. It is as if they spin around an axis like spinning tops. It is a fact of physics that they can live in one of only two states of spin, that we might call 'up' and 'down'. Atomic particles tend to pair up with each other, with one particle in the 'up' spin state and the other in the 'down'. The hydrogen atom is simply a proton, whose spin is therefore unpaired. Or 'unmarried', perhaps.

When a magnetic field is applied, the unpaired spins line up in it. In any given strength of magnetic field, it takes a precise amount of energy to flip the proton from one spin state to another. The proton, now 'spinning' the wrong way round for the field, flips back to its preferred orientation, a process called 'relaxation'. In this 'relaxation', energy is emitted in the form of a quantum of electromagnetic radiation, a photon, and it is this emitted energy which is picked up by the magnetic resonance scanner. *The rate of relaxation is highly dependent on the local chemical environment.*

The scanner looks at in two ways, 'T1' and 'T2'. The 'T' in these two refers to time that it takes for the energy to be emitted. T1 refers to relaxation along the line of the magnetic field, T2 to relaxation at right angles to it. T2 is a complex concept to get across, but T2 relaxation (and the associated energy emission) has to do with the spins falling out of synchrony with each other. There is a disordering, which emits energy.

The point about these two modes, T1 and T2, is that they give different 'takes' on the scan. T1 is especially useful for showing anatomy, while T2 is useful for showing water, and especially (in the technique known as FLAIR), 'pathological' water, being water that should not be there. In common with every other tissue, capillaries in damaged brain leak fluid, and MRI is especially good at picking this up.

2.7.2. The Neurological Dysfunctions

I have divided up the complex business of neurology into nine 'dysfunction syndromes' which are roughly anatomical (Table 2.7.2, Figure 2.7). These categories represent a simple way to start getting into neurology.

Perhaps the commonest neurological dysfunction is the upper motor neurone hemiplegia caused by **motor cortex** damage. Problems of the **frontal lobe** (and its 'connections') give 'thinking'-type problems, called 'cognitive'. The **basal ganglia** are associated with the initiation of movement (too little or too much). The **cerebellum** has to do with control of movement: damage to the cerebellum makes the patient clumsy, or 'ataxic'. The **brainstem** is a very important control centre where a small lesion can cause major disease, often with signs in the cranial nerves and a drop in conscious level. The **spinal cord** is sometimes subject to surgically-correctable compression and this situation can be an emergency. Cancer and trauma are common underlying pathologies here. The **peripheral nerves** are subject to metabolic deficiency or poisoning, and trauma. **Meningism**, irritation of the sensitive meningeal membranes, can be caused by infection or bleeding into the CSF. Lastly, **raised intracranial pressure** causes displacement of the brain within the skull, squeezing the brain stem down into the foramen magnum.

When neurological disease becomes very advanced, it is the respiratory and renal systems which are affected. Aspiration pneumonia occurs if the conscious level falls, or if there is severe muscular weakness or brain stem problems affecting the gag reflex, or simply causing hypoventilation. Urinary retention, with urinary infection and possibly renal dysfunction, are features of failure in the spinal cord and sometimes the peripheral nerves.

Treatment of neurological conditions depends very much on the syndrome, but there are generic supportive measures for neurology patients, described in Useful Box 2.35.

Table 2.7.2. Summary: Nine (Roughly) Anatomical Dysfunction Syndromes in Neurology.

	Name	*Main problem and signs*
1	Motor cortex	Contralateral upper motor neurone hemiplegia ± speech or visual defect. Weakness with increased tone, increased tendon reflexes, upgoing plantars. ± Homonymous hemianopia in fields.
2	Cognitive: mainly frontal lobe	Poor memory, disinhibited or otherwise altered personality. Assess by mental test score.
3	Basal ganglia	Movement disorder, especially with initiation of movement (too little or too much). Power is preserved. Tone often increased; with 'pill-rolling' tremor. Abnormal facial expression (blank in Parkinson's).
4	Cerebellum	Ataxia, nystagmus, incoordination, intention tremor. Past pointing.
5	Brainstem	Cranial nerves, conscious level, possibly 'long tract'. Examination of cranials especially III VI VII IIX IX X XI XII. Assess conscious level using Glasgow coma scale.
6	Spinal cord	Paraplegia, sensory level, bowels and bladder dysfunction. The idea of a 'level' above which things are normal but below, not.
7	Peripheral nerve	Glove and stocking sensory loss, ±motor weakness. Diminished power, flaccid tone, decreased reflexes, impaired sensation.
8	Raised intracranial pressure	Headache, vomiting, impaired conscious level, papilloedema. Conscious level (as for brainstem). Papilloedema, pupil size.
9	Meningeal	Headache, neck stiffness, photophobia. Straight leg raising.

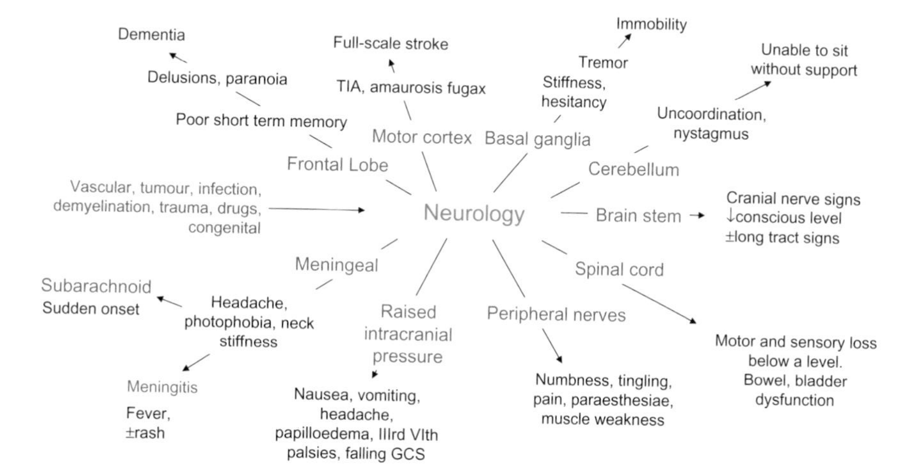

Figure 2.7. Different Neurological Dysfunction Syndromes. This map illustrates the nine different 'dimensions' that neurological disease can take. Any individual patient might follow one or possibly many of these arms, depending on the pathological process. For most of the arms, the further along the arm, the more severe the problem. For 'Meningeal' (bottom left), the two major illnesses, subarachnoid haemorrhage and meningitis, occur suddenly as emergencies and do not progress after admission, so I give simply the key features.

2.7.2.1. *Motor Cortex, Hemiplegia*

Motor weakness due to an upper motor neurone cortical lesion (Table 2.7.3) is the commonest of the neurological syndromes on a general medical ward. This prevalence reflects the susceptibility of the middle cerebral artery to blockage, probably because the middle cerebral is the largest branch of the internal carotid, and an ideal place for an embolus to go; a blockage here always leads to overt symptoms and signs. In addition to motor weakness, dysphasia or aphasia may be present, in which the patient cannot find the words to say what he or she wants. You will of course remember that the speech centre is on the left in all right-handed people, while in left-handed people, it can be on either side. A lesion affecting the motor cortex can also involve the optic radiations or even the occipital cortex, giving a contralateral hemianopia which you can easily test for. Patients do not understand the optic pathways (it's rusty for you too) and they will often report that they have 'a problem in the left eye', but it eventually turns out to be a left homonymous hemianopia, which of course affects both eyes. So do your tests well.

Useful Box 2.22. 'Upper and Lower Motor Neurone Signs'. This is a very useful diagnostic distinction in neurology. **Upper motor neurone**: increased tone with a springy, elastic feel; increased deep tendon reflexes, extensor plantar responses; and possibly, clonus. **Lower:** flaccid, floppy limbs. Muscle wasting and fasciculation. Decreased reflexes, flexor plantars.

Table 2.7.3. Motor Cortex.

Point	*Comment*
Classic features in a severe case	The key feature is unilateral weakness of one side of the body (i.e., 'hemiplegia'). Because it is an upper motor neurone condition (Useful Box 2.22), there is increased tone, increased deep tendon reflexes, an upgoing 'extensor' plantar, diminished abdominal reflexes, and sometimes clonus (Useful Box 2.23). Dysphasia or aphasia, depending on the side.
To look out for	'Dissection' of a carotid: sharp sudden pain up one side of the neck, with possible Horner's syndrome on that side. Caused by separation of the layers of the arterial wall.
Progression	In stroke, it usually tends to get at least a little better after the initial onset. In tumour, not.
Terminal events	Debility (i.e. weight loss, total body protein reduction, loss of muscle bulk and power, weakness, inability to clear chest secretions, reduced ability to fight infection, starved of proteins and energy). Chest infection. Bed sores and sepsis.
Likely causes	Cerebrovascular accident ('stroke') which can be thrombotic or haemorrhagic. Tumour.
Rare but treatable causes	Cerebral abscess. Traumatic extradural or subdural haemorrhage. Temporal arteritis.
Acute forms	Stroke.
Tests to be done	CT scan, typically followed by MRI. If the cause is stroke, cardiovascular investigations, including ECG and echo. Carotid Doppler (ultrasound of carotids), possibly MR angiogram of carotids.
Treatment	Thrombolytics are now being used for acute thrombotic stroke, but require major scanning and neurological support, for they must be used quickly after onset (<3 hours) and are not useful (indeed, dangerous) if the pathology is haemorrhagic. Dexamethasone if tumour is present.
Prognosis	Variable. Depends on initial lesion.

Useful Box 2.23. Clonus is a physical sign that can be elicited at either knee or ankle. At the knee, the patella is given a sharp shove down towards the feet; at the ankle, the foot is jerked sharply up to stretch the Achilles tendon. 'Clonus' occurs if the stretched muscle contracts and repetitively continues so to do after the stimulus.

2.7.2.2. *Cognitive: Mainly Frontal Lobe Dysfunction*

The frontal lobe (and connections) are to do with thinking (Table 2.7.4). In this clinical context, the word 'cognitive' has to do with 'thinking power': memory, organisation, paying attention and concentrating, problem solving, prioritisation, understanding, learning (tested by some kind of 'Mental Test Score': Useful Box 2.24). The frontal lobes are also to do with personality: mood, approach, cheerfulness (or not). In clinical medicine, by far the commonest abnormality in this area is dementia. 'Cognitive impairment' is a phrase used at the bedside as a code for 'dementia'.

Dementia is chronic and often associated with 'Lewy body' pathology (Useful Box 2.25). 'Acute confusional states' can arise in any patient. Causes might include drugs, ischaemia, infection or metabolic upset.

Useful Box 2.24. Tests of Cognitive Power. Many simple question/task lists have been devised to assess cognitive power. The GP scoring system is based on the following questions and tests: (i) tell the patient an address for recall in a minute or two; (ii) ask about today's date (iii) ask patient to draw a clock face; (iv) tell doc about an item of recent news; (v) ask about address given at the outset.

Useful Box 2.25. The Lewy Body. An insoluble deposit of alpha-synuclein in a neurone. A classic kind of neuronal pathology in which the very gradual accumulation of an insoluble protein in a cell impairs its function; dementia results. It's the problem of never being able to actually replace the cells with new ones. In other tissues, by and large, cells laden with unwanted protein can be replaced.

Table 2.7.4. Cognitive Dysfunction: Summary.

Point	*Comment*
Classic features in a severe case	'Cognitive function' (basically thinking) loss is the key event. Memory, attention, language and problem solving. First short-term memory is lost, then later longer-term memory. There can be changes in the personality: angry, truculent, difficult, perhaps weepy. Typically sullen, sometimes euphoric. Incontinence can develop and a susceptibility to absent-minded self-harm, leaving cooking rings on, or tripping and falling.
To look out for	Hypothyroidism, B_{12} deficiency.
Progression	Over years.
Terminal events	Quite often it's an accident: falling and fracturing a neck of femur.
Likely causes	Most cases in the elderly are idiopathic. Efforts are always made to exclude B_{12} deficiency and hypothyroidism but the hit rate is not high, it has to be said.
Rare but treatable causes	Subdural haematoma, hypercalcaemia, tumour, syphilis.
Acute forms	'Delirium' is the word: infection (e.g. streptococcal pneumonia in younger people, UTI in older patients), metabolic (e.g. hypoglycaemia, ethanol withdrawal).
Tests to be done	Functional assessment: the 'dementia screen'. CT head. Thyroid function. B_{12}, folate. EEG.
Treatment	Is mainly supportive. The prevention of harm, the maintaining of hygiene and human dignity are the major tasks of the medical team. The doctor's job is to diagnose, to treat intercurrent illnesses and to manage humanely.
Prognosis	The books say that it takes seven years to die after dementia first starts, and that's about right.

2.7.2.3. *Basal Ganglia Dysfunction*

The classic problem centred on the basal ganglia (Table 2.7.5) is Parkinson's disease. Motor power is preserved but the patient cannot use it effectively. Basal ganglia failure is not a problem of coordination or power but a problem of initiation of movement. There is a lack of voluntary movement, a slowness in getting going. Typically there is increased tone in the limbs, and a coarse (i.e. comparatively low frequency) tremor, which disappears when the patient concentrates on moving, and reappears when the patient is at rest. The facial expression tends to be blank. Reflexes are not abnormal.

The increase in tone is described as like a 'lead pipe'. The point is that when you try and flex or extend the patient's elbow, there is a constant resistance to the force that you apply. The joint will bend, and once you have stopped applying the force the joint will remain in the same position. This is in contrast to the increased tone in upper-motor-neurone lesions, where the resistance to your force varies in the arc and there is a springy quality about the bending.

We concentrate on Parkinson's here, but there are patients with a 'polar opposite' basal ganglia problem, where they have movements that are uncontrollably active. See Useful Box 2.26.

Parkinson's is treated with 'levo-dopa'. The drug, which is a derivative of the amino acid tyrosine, crosses the blood-brain barrier and is a precursor for the synthesis of dopamine (itself a precursor of noradrenaline and adrenaline, please note). The drug works because Parkinson's is caused by loss of dopamine-secreting cells. The levo-dopa is commonly combined with an inhibitor of dopa decarboxylase, which does not cross the blood-brain barrier, and prevents the conversion of the levo-dopa to catecholamines outside the brain.

Table 2.7.5. Basal Ganglia Dysfunction.

Point	*Comment*
Classic features in a severe case	A problem of initiation of movement rather than motor strength itself. There is hesitation in getting going, and the movement itself is unduly rapid and imperfectly controlled. Sensation and motor power are preserved. There is typically a pill-rolling tremor in which the index finger and thumb seem to move against each other to roll a particle between them.
To look out for	Occult malignancy. A Parkinsonian basal ganglia syndrome can be the immunologically-mediated result of a tumour in another system. This is called a 'paraneoplastic syndrome'.
Progression	Gradual over years.
Terminal events	Respiratory problems. Falls.
Likely causes	Vast majority of cases are 'idiopathic'. Drugs, especially anti-psychotics, can be a cause. Vascular.
Rare but treatable causes	Wilson's disease: young people only.
Acute forms	Drug-induced: phenothiazines.
Tests to be done	Brain scan. Wilson's disease tests, possibly.
Treatment	Levo-dopa with dopa decarboxylase inhibitor (levo-dopa is converted to catecholamines: the decarboxylase inhibitor, which does not cross the blood-brain barrier, stops this unwelcome peripheral conversion. It's cute). Others.
Prognosis	Not bad.

Useful Box 2.26. Other Basal Ganglia Problems Can Occur. Parkinson's is a *deficiency* in movement but some patients show excessive, uncontrollable movements which can take a number of different forms. The common causes of such excessive movement, known as 'chorea', athetosis' and 'tics', are treatment for Parkinson's, anti-psychotic drugs and a series of inherited conditions including Huntington's Chorea, which features in Ian McEwan's novel about UCH, 'Saturday'.

2.7.2.4. *Cerebellar Failure*

Cerebellar dysfunction (Table 2.7.6) is one of the two major effects of acute alcohol intoxication. The cerebellar patient staggers as if drunk, and is often falsely accused of being so. Cerebellar problems can easily be unilateral. (It's ipsilateral, by the way: left cerebellum gives signs on the left.)

Cerebellar problems are caused by cerebrovascular disease, tumours, multiple sclerosis, drugs.

The key clinical term is 'ataxia', meaning 'lack of order'. Movements are incoordinated. The patient shows an 'ataxic gait': staggering, often falling dangerously and is unable to lift a cup to the mouth effectively.

There is a really useful mnemonic to help you remember the main features of the cerebellar syndrome. It's 'DASHING':

- dysdiadochokinesis, clumsiness in repetitive movements;
- ataxia, staggering uncoordinated movements;
- speech;
- hypotonia, flaccidity at the joints;
- intention tremor, when the finger oscillates when trying to point to your finger;
- nystagmus, a repetitive jerking movements of the eyes;
- gait, which is staggering.

There is no specific pharmacological treatment for cerebellar disease, unfortunately.

Table 2.7.6. Cerebellar Dysfunction: Summary.

Point	*Comment*
Classic features in a severe case	'Ataxia': a loss of coordination. Staggering, unstable gait; as if drunk, without the euphoria (which is a frontal lobe effect). Difficulty in speaking. Motor power is preserved but the patient has difficulty in using it effectively. Reflexes are typically present and not brisk or reduced.
To look out for	Acoustic neuroma (benign tumour of the eighth cranial nerve, more precisely termed 'vestibular schwannoma'). Unilateral nerve deafness.
Progression	Depends on the cause.
Terminal events	As for hemiplegia.
Likely causes	Alcohol. Ischaemia. Drugs. Tumour. Demyelination. Inherited ataxia.
Rare but treatable causes	Wernicke's encephalopathy (see Useful Box 3.5). Hypothyroidism (see Section 2.6.2). Coeliac disease.
Acute forms	Drug induced (e.g. phenytoin); stroke.
Tests to be done	CT is not especially useful for the cerebellum: the MRI is much better.
Treatment	Treat the cause, if possible. Physio, psycho-social support, OT. Physical assistance: sticks, supports, wheelchairs, cars, mobility. See 'neuro support'.
Prognosis	Depends on the cause.

2.7.2.5. *Brainstem Dysfunction*

The brainstem is a very fundamental control centre packed with small but very important structures, most notably the control of respiration, consciousness and sleep. A lot of important tracts run up and down through it, too: sensory, motor and cerebellar (known as 'long tracts': Useful Box 2.27). So small lesions in the brain stem can cause major problems (e.g. Weber syndrome, Useful Box 2.28). The key to diagnosis here is the examination of the cranial nerves III–XII.

Table 2.7.7 shows the fundamental clinical aspects of brain stem disease. There will be some combination of change in cranial nerves III to XII (e.g. facial weakness, eye movement paralysis, pupillary asymmetry, tongue deviation) with or without a long tract abnormality (hemiplegia perhaps) and with or without a variation in conscious level.

There is an overlap between 'raised intracranial pressure' (Section 2.7.2.8) and 'brainstem', because raised intracranial pressure pushes the brain stem (with the cerebellar tonsils) down into the foramen magnum, compressing the stem, possibly inhibiting respiration (known as 'coning'). It is every doctor's nightmare, that one, I'll tell you.

Useful Box 2.27. 'Long Tract Signs' is a term used by neurologists to describe motor and/or sensory signs in the limbs or trunk due to involvement of the cable bundles running up and down through the brain stem. Obviously you have to know the levels of the decussations. Upper motor neurons and dorsal columns (vibration, position) cross over in the medulla, while the spinothalamic tract (touch, temperature) crosses at the level of entry to the cord.

Table 2.7.7. Brainstem Dysfunction.

Point	*Comment*
Classic features in a severe case	Clouding of consciousness. Cranial nerve signs, 'long tract' signs. Pontine disease gives pinpoint pupils and unconsciousness. Can see dysarthria, facial weakness, facial numbness and disordered extra-ocular movements.
To look out for	Easily confused with increased intracranial pressure.
Progression	Very variable.
Terminal events	Apnoea, aspiration, cardiac arrest.
Likely causes	Ischaemia. Demyelination.
Rare but treatable causes	Central pontine myelinolysis after rapid changes in metabolic conditions (plasma Na, others) is said to be avoidable if not perhaps easily treatable. Sarcoid and TB are treatable.
Acute forms	Ischaemia, coning.
Tests to be done	MRI is especially useful. LP sometimes.
Treatment	Underlying cause. May have to paralyse, intubate and ventilate to protect the airway. Nasogastric (or PEG) feeding.
Prognosis	Not typically good.

Useful Box 2.28. 'Weber syndrome'. Nowhere is neuroanatomy more important than in brainstem neurology. The very detailed apposition of long tracts and nuclei comes into play. For instance, a 'Weber's syndrome' is the occurrence of an ipsilateral oculomotor palsy with a contralateral hemiplegia. This is caused by a lesion at the level of the midbrain, impinging on the IIIrd nucleus and the descending motor tract, not yet crossed over. There are many other such named syndromes in brainstem neurology.

2.7.2.6. *Spinal Cord Dysfunction*

Spinal cord *compression* may be treatable by surgery and is a vital clinical diagnosis. It's a true emergency, since if there is pressure on the cord itself (as opposed to the *cauda equina*, see below) the extent of subsequent recovery strongly depends on how quickly the compression is relieved. It is said that if the compression is sufficient to cause complete paralysis, then a delay of more than 24 hours is associated only rarely with a good recovery.

The key features of spinal cord dysfunction are shown in Table 2.7.8. It depends on the exact location of the problem, but the patient presents with some kind of combination of sensory problems in the legs and feet, weakness of the legs and difficulty with bladder and bowel function. In your history you will be keen to get clues about such underlying diagnoses as trauma, cancer, slipped disc. Examination is key. You need to be as precise as you can about motor weakness, and about the actual extent and severity of sensory losses. The key finding in your examination is the identification of a 'level', below which things are abnormal, and above which all is well.

A lateralised lesion on one side of the cord gives the 'Brown-Séquard syndrome: Useful Box 2.29.

The key investigation is MRI. CT is okay, but not nearly as helpful as MRI. The nearby bones cast shadows which lessen the clarity of the CT images.

Useful Box 2.29. The Brown-Séquard Syndrome. One unusual but instructive spinal cord compression variant is the Brown-Séquard syndrome, where a small laterally-placed lesion picks out the motor and sensory nerve bundles on one side only. The upper motor neurone loss and the deficit in position and vibration sense are on the side of the lesion. The loss of temperature touch and pinprick sensation are on the other side, all below the level of the lesion. Brown-Séquard worked in London but was born in Mauritius.

Table 2.7.8. Spinal Cord Dysfunction.

Point	*Comment*
Classic features in a severe case	We'll say that the compression is at T10. Symmetrical weakness of the legs, numbness of the lower limbs and trunk to level of T10, usually symmetrical but see 'Brown-Séquard' Box 2.29. Symptoms relating to difficulty with bowels and bladder.
To look out for	This condition, itself. It sounds like a simple diagnosis but it is one that you will not see often and you do have to think of it, to ask yourself the question, 'Has this patient got spinal cord compression?'
Progression	Unpredictable.
Terminal events	Renal failure can result from obstruction to drainage of bladder. Bed sores can become infected. Some patients, confined to wheelchairs and not in control of bowels and bladder, are suicidal. Many of these patients have cancer in the first place.
Likely causes	Cancer. Prolapsed disc. Demyelination. Ischaemia. Trauma.
Rare but treatable causes	I once read of a case where the spinal cord compression was due to an accumulation of cholesterol near the cord.
Acute forms	Frequently acute. Cancer, trauma, prolapsed intervertebral disc, ischaemia.
Tests to be done	MRI scan of the spine. The CT is not so useful because the enclosing bony spinal column causes shadows. The MRI shows not only abnormal anatomy but also demyelination, if present. CT does not show this pathology.
Treatment	Can be surgery, and quickly too. Catheterise. Dexamethasone, as for raised ICP.
Prognosis	Varies, from complete recovery to permanent paralysis.

2.7.2.7. *Peripheral Nerve Dysfunction*

A gradual failure of the peripheral nerves is often seen in diabetes and alcoholism (Table 2.7.9). The key feature in failure of the peripheral nerves is bilateral glove-and-stocking sensory loss, sometimes with pins and needles and pain. The longest nerves tend to be affected first, so that the feet and hands are the earliest areas to show symptoms and signs. Some forms, especially the rapid Guillain-Barré form, predominantly affect the motor nerves.

Aside from the symmetrical glove-and-stocking peripheral neuropathy that we consider here, there are very many peripheral nerve and nerve root problems in neurology, often caused by pressure on the nerve or direct trauma to it. Two important conditions that affect peripheral nerves in special ways, motor neurone disease and myasthenia gravis, are considered in Useful Box 2.30. A genetic form of peripheral neuropathy is discussed in Useful Box 2.31.

Useful Box 2.30. Motor Neurone Disease and Myasthenia Gravis.

Motor neurone disease is a slowly progressive condition of both upper and lower motor neurones. Lower motor neurone failure is shown by muscle wasting and fasciculation (a flickering random contraction in recently denervated muscle). Upper motor neurone failure is shown by a tendency to hypertonia and increased reflexes, especially in the more proximal muscles. Thus one can see increased reflexes and clonus at the knee, with absent ankle jerks (lower motor neurone) and extensor plantar responses (upper motor neurone).

Myasthenia gravis is another motor weakness disease but its pathology and clinical picture are different from motor neurone disease. Caused by antibodies to the acetylcholine receptor, the picture of myasthenia is of variable severity of weakness, typically worse after repeated use of the muscle, and often presenting with diplopia. It can be treated with anticholinesterase drugs which prolong the presence of acetylcholine at the motor end-plate.

Table 2.7.9. Peripheral Nerve Dysfunction.

Point	*Comment*
Classic features in a severe case	Pain and numbness in the feet and later the hands. Wasting, with weakness of the muscles in the legs and feet. Diminished sensation to light touch in a glove and stocking pattern. Weakness in muscles, possibly with fasciculation. Diminished deep tendon reflexes especially in the ankles. Symptoms and signs can ascend until finally respiration is compromised.
To look out for	B_{12} deficiency. Multiple myeloma.
Progression	Typically very gradual.
Terminal events	Respiratory compromise. Uncontrollable aspiration pneumonia. Renal infection and/or obstructive renal failure.
Likely causes	Diabetes, ethanol.
Rare but treatable causes	B_{12} deficiency; syphilis; AIDS.
Acute forms	Guillain-Barré: a predominantly motor autoimmune peripheral neuropathy. Young patient; 'ascending paralysis'; high protein level in CSF.
Tests to be done	Studies of nerve conduction are useful to confirm diagnosis of neuropathy. Blood count, B_{12} level, protein electrophoresis.
Treatment	'Supportive', sometimes to the extent of assisted ventilation. The patient with diminished sensation needs expert nursing care to prevent pressure sores. Physiotherapy helps to keep joints moving during neurological inactivity.
Prognosis	Depends strongly on the cause. Can be very debilitating, but most cases are not so bad, typically. A nuisance and a problem rather than a terminal event.

Useful Box 2.31. Charcot-Marie-Tooth disease. This is one of the most common inherited neurological conditions. There are many variations on the main theme, but most cases are inherited as autosomal dominants (both sexes, direct transmission from generation to generation). There is a gradual deterioration in motor and sensory function in the peripheral nerves. The feet are affected first, in true 'peripheral neuropathy' fashion. There is wasting of muscle, with imbalance between flexors and extensors, which leads to deformity.

2.7.2.8. *Raised Intracranial Pressure*

Raised intracranial pressure (Table 2.7.10) can result from tumour, intracranial haemorrhage, abscess, thrombosis in a venous sinus, metabolic upset or obstruction to the drainage of CSF. Many of these are surgically remediable. It is obviously very important to be able to recognise this syndrome.

It is not an easy diagnosis. You are unlikely to see it often. Apart from papilloedema, there are no really characteristic signs. The diagnosis of papilloedema requires firstly that you can find a working ophthalmoscope, and secondly that you can use it effectively. It is a great help to have seen a handful of cases of papilloedema before. You can see how the difficulties are mounting up. Deteriorating conscious level is an important clinical sign which can be assessed by the Glasgow coma scale (Useful Box 2.32).

The classic brain tumour picture is of incessant headache, worse in the mornings, with anorexia and possibly vomiting. The patient may be noted to be increasingly sleepy. On examination it might be noted that the blood pressure is high while the pulse is slow. There may be abnormalities in cranial nerves III and VI. The pupils may be dilated.

The real-life intracranial pressure diagnostic problem is likely to be challenging: a smelly abusive drunk with a head wound and slightly unequal pupils, which might have been like that for decades.

The CT scan is invaluable. It does not actually measure the pressure directly, but it will show you if there is a 'space-occupying lesion' (tumour, haemorrhage, abscess) or CSF blockage inside the skull. If there is no lesion visible then it is unlikely that there will be a useful surgical intervention.

Dexamethasone is an invaluable short-term holding treatment to try and alleviate the cerebral oedema that often accompanies acute brain lesions. The patient may have to be ventilated.

Table 2.7.10. Raised Intracranial Pressure.

Point	*Comment*
Classic features in a severe case	Headache, nausea, vomiting, drowsiness, papilloedema, slow pulse, high BP, abnormal respiratory pattern sixth and/or third nerve paralysis, dilated pupils, seizures, respiratory depression, death.
To look out for	The diagnosis itself.
Progression	Can be slow or rapid depending on underlying pathology.
Terminal events	Respiratory depression.
Likely causes	Tumour, primary or secondary; haemorrhage. Oedema often plays a significant part. Infection.
Rare but treatable causes	Intracranial venous sinus thrombosis. Hyperammonaemia of liver failure.
Acute forms	Trauma, giving intracranial haemorrhage.
Tests to be done	CT brain; possibly MRI if CT is normal.
Treatment	Dexamethasone or mannitol to reduce pressure. Maintain ventilation, avoid hypoxia (may need respiratory support.) Often, surgery and/or radiotherapy. Anticonvulsants if necessary.
Prognosis	Variable. Depending on the cause and the speed of treatment (one element of which is the time it takes you to make the diagnosis, so read this, digest it and be ready).

Useful Box 2.32. The Glasgow Coma Scale is a very useful way of monitoring conscious level. The scale is based on three clinical assessments. Eye opening, from spontaneous opening (4 points) to no response (1 point); verbal response: from normal conversation (5 points) to ‘no sound’ (1 point); and ‘best motor response’, from obeying commands perfectly (6 points) to no movement (1 point). The maximum score is 15 (minimum possible is 3). Once the patient gets down to 8 or less, intubation and ventilation become desirable.

2.7.2.9. *Meningism*

'Meningism' (Table 2.7.11), meaning the combination of headache, photophobia and stiffness of the neck (basically, resistance to flexion), is an important syndrome in medicine, possibly pointing as it does to two very serious conditions: bacterial meningitis, which is infection in the CSF irritating the meninges, or subarachnoid haemorrhage (Useful Box 2.33), which is a bleed from an artery in the circle of Willis into the CSF. It is a curious fact that the substance of the brain is essentially anaesthetic: in spite of all the neurones that are there, there are no pain receptors. But the meninges are very well equipped with pain receptors, and chemical or inflammatory irritation of the meninges, or stretching of them, is sensitively appreciated as pain. Blood, as in SAH, causes a chemical irritation.

The actual symptoms of meningism are not an uncommon finding, and happily only a minority of cases have either of the two major diagnoses above.

If you seriously suspect bacterial meningitis then it is reasonable, indeed essential, to give antibiotics without further delay. Otherwise, you have time to get a CT and then an LP.

'Meningism' is not always caused by these two unpleasant diseases. *Viral* meningitis is considered in Useful Box 2.34. Obviously headache is a very common symptom. Headache combined with photophobia and stiffness of the neck can occur in migraine and even in 'tension headache', and in a number of feverish illnesses that do not involve the meninges... but since it is very bad to miss bacterial meningitis or SAH, we end up doing many negative LPs. It's life. There is no other way, at present.

Useful Box 2.33. The Subarachnoid Haemorrhage is a leak from a 'berry aneurysm', a congenital dilatation in the circle of Willis, often located at a branch point. It is not of atheromatous pathology. Subarachnoid is a disease of younger patients.

Table 2.7.11. Meningism: Summary.

Point	*Comment*
Classic features in a severe case	Headache, neck stiffness, photophobia, difficult straight-leg raise. In bacterial meningitis, onset is over days or at least hours, and there is fever. In meningococcal meningitis, famous non-blanching skin rash. In sub-arachnoid, very sudden 'thunderclap' onset, typically no fever. Can be papilloedema.
To look out for	The rash.
Progression	Depends on the cause.
Terminal events	(In infection) septic shock (see Section 2.11). Brain damage, cardiac arrest.
Likely causes	For infection, *Neiserria meningitidis*, *Streptococcus pneumoniae*, some others. For subarachnoid, berry aneurysm.
Rare but treatable causes	It is occasionally traumatic in origin: a tear in the meninges.
Acute forms	It's all acute here.
Tests to be done	CT brain; lumbar puncture; bloods. MR very useful in SAH, to show vessels.
Treatment	Depends on the cause. Urgent antibiotics for meningitis, obviously.
Prognosis	Very variable.

Useful Box 2.34. Viral Meningitis. Often caused by enteroviruses, 'viral meningitis' is typically a much less severe illness than bacterial meningitis. The symptoms are similar, if perhaps slower in onset and generally milder. The lumbar puncture gives clear fluid with lymphocytes as the abnormal cell type and there is of course no growth on bacterial culture. There is no treatment, unless *Herpes simplex* is suspected, in which case the anti-viral aciclovir can be given.

2.7.3. Intersections in Neurology

Table 2.7.12 shows the *common* ways in which the pathological processes (as they occur in neurology (Section 2.7.1)) apply to the anatomical dysfunction syndromes that we have just discussed.

The point is that some pathologies selectively affect different parts of the nervous system. Cancer within the skull can affect any of cortex, basal ganglia, cerebellum and stem, but mostly it is motor cortex, frontal cortex and cerebellum where the signs show. Malignant pressure on spinal cord from tumours in the vertebral bodies is common. MS can affect only the central nervous system and not peripheral nerves. The main autoimmune condition of the peripheral nerves is Guillain-Barré syndrome (they were French).

There are very many congenital neurological conditions. Perinatal hypoxia is unfortunately still quite common, and like all other systems there are accidents in development, notably inadequate fusion of the neural tube, giving 'spina bifida' and the picture of spinal cord dysfunction.

Table 2.7.12. Summary of the Main Intersections in Neurology.

	Pathological Process							
	Vascular	*Infection*	*Metabolic*	*Tumour*	*Inflammatory*	*Congenital*	*Trauma*	*Drug*
Dysfunction								
Motor cortex	Stroke	Abscess, encephalitis		Primary, secondary	MS	Cerebral palsy	Subdural, extradural hh	
Frontal lobe	Vascular dementia	Abscess, encephalitis	Alzheimers, hypothyroid	Primary, secondary	MS	Cerebral palsy	Subdural, extradural hh	Alcohol, Steroids
Basal ganglia		—	Parkinson's	Primary, secondary	MS	Huntington's		Anti-psychotics
Cerebellum	Cerebellar stroke	—	Ethanol	Primary, secondary	MS	Inherited ataxias		Alcohol
Brainstem	Brainstem stroke	TB-	Wernicke's		MS, sarcoid			Opiates
Spinal cord	Ischaemic myelopathy	Pressure from abscess outside cord		Cord compression	MS	Spina bifida	Spinal column fracture	
Peripheral nerve	—	—	Diabetes, B_{12} defic		Guillain-Barré	Charcot-Marie-Tooth	Limb trauma	Anti-TB drugs
Raised intra-cranial pressure	SAH, venous sinus thrombosis	Abscess	—	Primary, secondary			Subdural, extradural hh	
Meningism	SAH	Meningitis	—				Torn dura	

Useful Box 2.35. 'Neurological Support'

Many of the conditions described in this neurology section culminate in a chronically-disabled patient whose major problem is some form of motor weakness. There may be cognitive and sensory problems, but an inability to move with power renders the patient more or less helpless in an especially tragic way. There are supportive measures that can be initiated to help the patient manage as best he or she can.

Nursing

- Administer medication if needed.
- Ensure hygiene and care of the skin, especially if anaesthetic.
- Intermittent catheterisation, if necessary.
- Manual evacuation of rectum, if necessary.
- Care of PEG tube if present.
- Stockings to prevent DVT in immobile limbs.

Occupational Therapy

- Wheelchair.
- Home modifications on the lines of disability access.
- Ensure safety of patient if memory is poor.
- Car adaptation if necessary.

Physiotherapy

- Maintain passive mobility of joints. Optimise mobility.
- Chest physio if needed.

Speech and Language

- Assess swallowing ability (thickened fluids required?).

Dietician

- Thickened fluids if required.
- Ensure adequate fluid and food intake.
- Dietary fibre content.

All Specialists

- Psychological aspects of the condition. Patient and family need support here.

2.8. RHEUMATOLOGICAL FAILURE

The joints are one of the two classic targets for autoimmune disease, the endocrine glands being the other. The commonest rheumatological diagnosis is 'rheumatoid arthritis' (Table 2.8, Figure 2.8) but there are many others (Box 2.37). The patient is typically a female of 20–45. The joints are hot, swollen, painful ('inflamed', obviously) and stiff, they do not work well, and can end up more or less destroyed. There is an associated inflammatory state in the body, a 'systemic inflammatory reaction', manifest as a high CRP, high ESR, normochromic anaemia with a low iron and low iron binding capacity, and a low albumin (exactly what is seen in chronic infection). Sometimes auto-antibodies can be found in the blood, notably 'rheumatoid factor'. There can be problems in other systems: often it is renal failure. There is weight loss. The exact diagnosis may not be clear at first, but very often anti-inflammatory drugs are the treatment.

The problems that you must deal with are the underlying inflammation, and then the resulting pain, stiffness and weakness. The treatment typically involves some form of immunosuppression. The blood tests are a useful adjunct to the patient's symptoms in assessing what treatment is required. The treatment may have to be quite intense and you can find yourself going down the immune deficiency pathway (Section 2.10).

'Support' in all its forms is needed for these chronically ill patients. Optimism can flag. The constant pain gets them down, quite apart from the limitations on mobility. They need help from physiotherapists and occupational therapists to keep the joints flexible and to optimise movement (comparable to the chronically neurologically ill, Useful Box 2.35). Surgery, including joint replacement (big joints only right now), can help a great deal.

Under Rheumatology we should consider 'vasculitis', that accompanies many autoimmune conditions. See Useful Box 2.36.

Table 2.8. Rheumatoid Failure.

Point	*Comment*
Classic features in a severe case	A woman in her forties starts with small joints that are stiff and painful in the mornings. Untreated, the problem worsens, spreads to other joints, causes chronic pain and harms the joints, resulting in the dislocation, erosion and stiffening of joints. May or may not be signs of disease in other systems. Osteoporosis is common.
To look out for	Vasculitic problems: a spotty purpuric rash, proteinuria, increasing creatinine.
Progression	Typically chronic with relapses and remissions.
Terminal events	Premature vascular disease. Debility from wasting of muscles.
Likely causes	Autoimmune: as rheumatoid arthritis, systemic lupus erythematosus, psoriasis-related arthropathy.
Rare but treatable causes	'Septic arthritis', i.e. bacterial infection within the joint capsule. Often requires surgical drainage.
Acute forms	Post-infective: widespread joint inflammation can occur after infections distant to the joints, especially diarrhoeal illnesses.
Tests to be done	FBC, ESR, CRP. Rheumatoid factor and other rheumatologically-related autoantibodies such as ANCA and ANF. X-rays of joints.
Treatment	Immunosuppression. B-cell depletion. Anti-TNF antibodies or other TNF-suppressing medications.
Prognosis	Variable.

Useful Box 2.36. Vasculitis. As part of rheumatology we should consider one of the most conceptually difficult forms of disease: vasculitis. The name itself means 'inflammation of blood vessels'. So what? Hot, tender blood vessels? Sometimes, but only if larger vessels are involved: usually, it is only smaller vessels that are affected. Vessels blocked by swollen walls? That's more like it. Vessel walls weakened and leaking by dint of inflammatory infiltrate of destructive immune cells throwing their weight around where they are not wanted? That happens too. Vasculitis is most often autoimmune in origin. Direct bacterial infection can very rarely do it, syphilis being the classic example. There is a ranking order for susceptibility to vasculitic attack: skin (most common)> kidney> brain> limbs> gut> lung> heart. Arthritis occurs in many vasculitic conditions, especially systemic lupus erythematosus and sometimes in rheumatoid arthritis.

At present it is treated with immunosuppressants in much the same way as auto-immune arthritis.

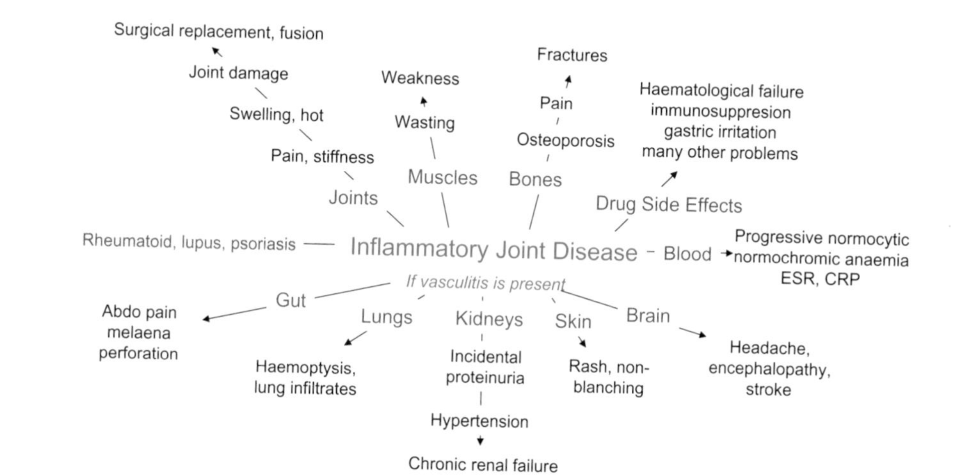

Figure 2.8. Map: The Patient with Inflammatory Joint Disease. This figure summarises the problems of the patient with 'active', autoimmune joint problems, typified by rheumatoid arthritis. The top half illustrates the progressions in joints, muscles, bones and drug side effect problems that can occur. The lower half of the figure illustrates the problems that can occur if the troublesome pathology of 'vasculitis' is part of the disease. The main targets for vasculitis are skin and kidneys, but in theory any tissue can be affected.

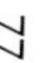

Useful Box 2.37. The Common Diseases of the Musculoskeletal System.

Ankylosing Spondylitis is an autoimmune disease, typically of young men who carry the HLA type B27. It affects the spine, causing pain and eventually much stiffness.

Gout is a monoarticular disease that tends to affect one or at most a few joints, very commonly the big toe. Gout is a metabolic disease, not autoimmune, caused by precipitation of crystals of sodium urate within the joint. The crystals cause an intense inflammatory reaction.

Osteoarthrosis is a 'mechanical' problem with joints. 'Wear and tear' describes it well. It comes to us all in our older years. Obesity accelerates its progress especially in the hips and knees. There is no autoimmunity with associated inflammatory reaction here.

Psoriatic Arthropathy is the arthritis that can go with the autoimmune skin disease known as psoriasis. The arthritis has a similar picture to rheumatoid, but the antibodies are negative (it is 'sero-negative').

Scleroderma ('Systemic Sclerosis') is an unusual autoimmune condition affecting the skin (which becomes tightened and contracted), oesophagus (likewise), joints (why found in this section), lungs, heart and kidney.

Septic Arthritis is a bacterial infection of a single joint. The bacteria usually get there via the blood. It is seen in injecting drug addicts who are not famed for the obsessiveness of their sterile technique.

Systemic Lupus Erythematosus (SLE, 'lupus') is a feared automimmune disease with a large vasculitic element. Anti-DNA antibodies are found in the blood.

2.9. HAEMATOLOGICAL FAILURE

By 'haematological failure' (Table 2.9) we mean failure of the bone marrow, failure to make its main products; red cells, white cells and platelets. There are a number of forms of this. It can be caused by malignant infiltration e.g. one of the leukaemias or multiple myeloma (a B-cell proliferation), or by drugs, usually chemotherapy for malignancy in other organs, by ionising radiation (as in 'whole body irradiation'), or by fibrotic infiltration as in myelofibrosis. Infections can cause it. There are autoimmune forms of 'aplastic anaemia'.

Figure 2.9 compares the main symptoms and signs arising from lack of the bone marrow products. Very severe shortage of red cells (that is, 'severe anaemia') makes the patient short of breath, drowsy and sometimes confused. Lack of neutrophils typically equals bacterial infection: a *very* low neutrophil count (less than about $0.5 \times 10^9/l$) renders the patient susceptible to aggressive infection by bacteria (so called 'neutropenic sepsis') and, over a longer time span, infection with the common fungus *Aspergillus fumigatus.* Lack of lymphocytes, as in AIDS, leads to different infections (see section 2.10, and Useful Box 2.39). When the platelet count falls very low ($<$about $20 \times 10^9/l$) spontaneous bleeding can occur.

The diagnosis is made by examination of the peripheral blood and later of the bone marrow. Radiology may show bony abnormalities suggesting a malignant process affecting the marrow. In deciding on treatment it is, as usual, important to try and identify the basic cause and then do something about it. 'Supportive' treatment in this haematological context consists of transfusion of blood products. Red cell transfusion is highly effective, but platelet transfusion is useful for only 24 hours at most.

Some important haematological conditions are considered in Useful Box 2.38.

Table 2.9. Haematological Failure.

Point	*Comment*
Classic features in a severe case	Failure of the bone marrow comes in many forms, acute and chronic, selective for cell types, or not. The patient can suffer from a combination of three main problems: weakness, fatigue, dyspnoea with red cell deficiency (ie 'anaemia'); a susceptibility to bacterial infection when the neutrophil count falls very low ('neutropenic sepsis'); and easy bruising or spontaneous bleeding when the platelets fall ('thrombocytopenia', 'thrombocytopenic purpura').
To look out for	Drug causes, which are potentially reversible. Uncontrolled infection.
Progression	Can obviously be very rapid indeed.
Terminal events	Massive sepsis, haemorrhage (from platelet deficiency), anaemia.
Likely causes	Drug-induced (chemotherapy, idiosyncratic reaction to another drug type); malignant infiltration of the marrow (leukaemia, myeloma, other); autoimmune; infection; fibrotic replacement of the marrow ('myelofibrosis').
Rare but treatable causes	Radiation poisoning. Social history may reveal that the patient is a KGB agent and has been poisoned with polonium-210 by his former colleagues (true UCH story!)
Acute forms	Chemotherapy, radiation.
Tests to be done	The blood count tells so much. Bone marrow biopsy may be needed. X-rays of bones containing marrow (skull, spine, femora) can be useful.
Treatment	Often chemotherapy is suspended while the marrow recovers. In neutropenia, intravenous broad spectrum antibiotics, given 'blindly' without bacteriological data, are often essential. Red cell and platelet transfusions are often necessary.
Prognosis	Variable. Not the happiest of diagnoses, it has to be said.

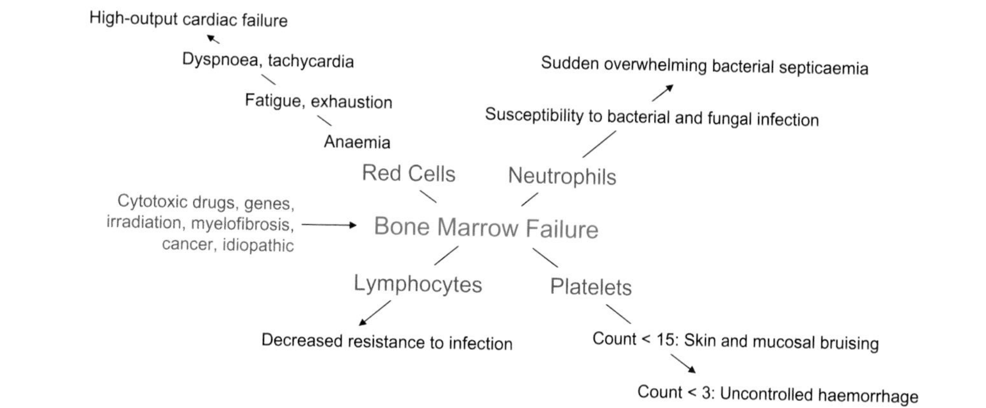

Figure 2.9. Map: Haematological Failure. This map illustrates the main problems seen in haematological failure. The basic pathology can affect all or only a subset of the pathways shown. 'Aplastic anaemia' would affect all four, while something like 'pure red cell aplasia' would (as it says) affect only red cells. This map focuses on lack of development but both red cells and platelets can be destroyed prematurely by antibodies in the circulation. Red cell manufacture is highly dependent on iron, vitamins including B_{12} and folate, and erythropoietin.

Useful Box 2.38. The Major Conditions and Diseases in Haematology.

Anaemia. A shortage of red cells can be caused by: bone marrow failure (occupation by malignancy or fibrosis); shortage of necessary building blocks (iron, B12, folate, others); lack of erythropoietin (renal failure); chronic inflammation (part of the 'acute phase response'); inherited red cell defects (alpha or beta globin mutations, many other genes, often associated with protection against malaria); destruction in the circulation by auto-antibodies ('autoimmune haemolytic anaemia').

Leukaemia. A malignant proliferation of cells forming neutrophils ('myeloid leukaemia') or lymphocytes ('lymphocytic leukaemia'). Can be 'acute' or 'chronic'. Acute myeloid is the most aggressive; chronic lymphocytic, the least aggressive.

Multiple Myeloma is a proliferation of plasma cells, which usually make and secrete into the blood a 'monoclonal' antibody. The quantity of this antibody can become very high and cause grief in the circulation, plugging glomeruli in particular.

Lymphoma is a malignant proliferation of lymphocytes. By and large the cells remain confined to the marrow, liver, spleen and lymph nodes but they can easily break out.

Immune Thrombocytopenic Purpura (ITP) is a classic autoimmune condition where the immune system makes antibodies against platelets. The count can be cut so low that spontaneous bleeding can occur.

Myelofibrosis is a slowly-progressive condition of older people in which fibrotic tissue takes over the marrow, reducing the space available for normal haematopoiesis. The spleen can become very much enlarged.

Haemochromatosis is a condition of iron overload. Physiological regulation of the iron content of the body occurs at the stage of absorption. There is no excretory pathway: neither the liver nor the kidneys can get rid of excess iron. In haemochromatosis there is an inherited abnormality in the absorptive process. Iron overload can also occur in many aggressive inherited haemolytic anaemias such as severe thalassaemias.

Clotting Problems such as haemophilia and von Willebrand's disease are a major part of haematology.

2.10. IMMUNODEFICIENCY

Any very ill and debilitated patient (undernourished perhaps, or with a major system failure), or any patient with an anatomical abnormality (e.g. a stone in a kidney) or a functional abnormality (e.g. a neurological patient with bladder dysfunction) becomes susceptible to infection. Diabetics are also at risk. The lack of a spleen is dangerous (Useful Box 2.4.1).

However, there are patients with normal anatomy and neurological function who suffer infections by virtue of defects in the immune defence system itself. Immunodeficiency can be congenital or acquired; it can be due to problems with neutrophils, T or B lymphocytes, or simply the amount of immunoglobulin in the plasma (summarized in Table 2.10 and Figure 2.10).

'Neutropenic' patients and those with 'antibody'-based immunodeficiency typically develop bacterial infections, which can be very aggressive in neutropenia. In 'cellular' immunodeficiencies, the T cells fail, giving a susceptibility to viral and protozoal infection.

A number of pathological processes can disrupt immune function. The chemotherapy for malignancy very often causes neutropenia, while steroids cause a T-cell defect. Secretion of immunoglobulins can be congenitally defective, or they can be lost through leaky glomeruli in the 'nephrotic syndrome'.

Easily the commonest cause of immunodeficiency worldwide is AIDS, in which the HIV virus disables the so-called 'CD4+ T lymphocyte', a form of lymphocyte which is key to the 'cell-mediated immunity' cascade. See Useful Box 2.39.

The presentation of immunodeficiency is typically with infection, although autoimmunity and cancer can occur (Useful Box 2.40).

Treatment will usually have two arms, one aimed at the attacking infection, the other aimed at the cause of the immunodeficiency, if it is possible to do anything about it: highly active anti-retroviral therapy for AIDS is very effective.

Table 2.10. Immunodeficiency.

Point	*Comment*
Classic features in a severe case	Obviously, unexpected infection is the classic problem, but it is usually the nature of the infection that flags up immunodeficiency. Pneumocystis, toxoplasmosis, cryptococcus, all occur in AIDS and pharmacological immunosuppression. Acute fever, often without a cause ever being found, is seen in neutropenia.
To look out for	This is dangerous, unpredictable, random territory. In AIDS and immunosuppression, you typically have some time (e.g. days) to make a diagnosis but in neutropenia (neutrophil count, less than about 0.5×10^9/l) things can move very quickly.
Progression	Very unpredictable. Antibiotics are terrific but a functioning immune system remains a very useful defensive system.
Terminal events	Overwhelming infection; malignancy.
Likely causes	HIV is commonest worldwide; chemotherapy; immunosuppression; congenital. The spleen has a defence role: splenectomy can be associated with rampant bacterial sepsis (see Useful Box 2.41).
Rare but treatable causes	In nephrotic syndrome immunoglobulins are lost in the urine.
Acute forms	Neutropenic sepsis.
Treatment	Firstly, you need treatment for the infection. Secondly, you can try and do something about the immunodeficiency. For AIDS, 'highly active retroviral therapy' is extremely useful. This consists of a combination of anti-retroviral medications, which inhibit such processes as the multiplication of retroviruses and the activity of HIV-1 protease.
Tests to be done	In HIV, the viral antibody, the viral load, and the CD4 count are the key tests for the infection; white cell count in the FBC; immunoglobulin levels; diagnosis of the opportunistic infection: CXR, scans, blood tests, biopsies — the whole gamut.
Prognosis	Very hard to predict. But by virtue of a massive amount of research, the prognosis of HIV in particular is much better than it was in 1982.

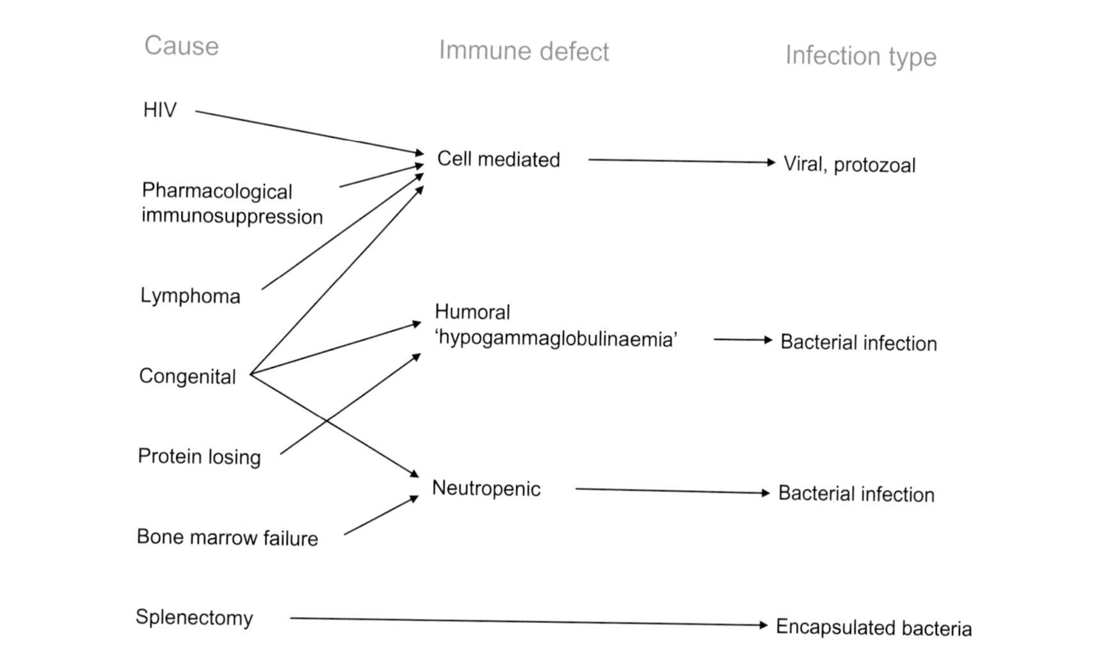

Figure 2.10. Immunodeficiency: Summary. Viruses, drugs, genes, protein-losing states (e.g. nephrotic syndrome), bone marrow failure and splenectomy can all cause forms of immunodeficiency. The immune defect can be in T-lymphocytes, B lymphocytes and immunoglobulins, in numbers or function of neutrophils, or in the filtering action of the spleen.

Useful Box 2.39. Common 'Opportunistic' Infections in AIDS.

Cytomegalovirus infection can easily occur in non-immunocompromised patients, but is responsible for lung, gut, retinal, liver, adrenal and neuronal problems in HIV.

Cryptococcosis, caused by the fungus *Cryptococcus neoformans,* which can give a mixture of these three components: meningitis, with a low grade fever and incessant headache; pulmonary cryptococcosis (a bilateral pneumonia picture) and cutaneous cryptococcosis, a papulo-nodular rash.

Kaposi Sarcoma, a malignant process giving purplish patches on the skin and other organs including the mouth, is itself caused by a herpes virus.

Oesophageal Candidiasis. Thrush in the oesophagus. Not typically a massive clinical problem, in that it does not kill the patient, but the fact is that candidiasis should never be in the oesophagus in an immunocompetent patient.

Pneumocystis Pneumonia. Fever, more fever, dry cough, dyspnoea, low arterial saturation, bilateral diffuse abnormality on the CXR.

Toxoplasmosis. In immunodeficients, causes brain abscesses, easily seen on the enhanced CT.

Useful Box 2.40. Wiskott-Aldrich Syndrome. This is a very rare, inherited immunodeficiency of children. It is caused by mutations in a cytoskeletal protein that acts as an anchor for actin filaments. The syndrome includes not only immunodeficiency but also autoimmunity and malignancy, illustrating the link between these three areas of medicine.

2.11. MAJOR SEPSIS

Infection is of course a very common form of human disease, and can take on a multiplicity of forms. Infections can have helpful specific diagnostic symptoms, signs and tests but we do not have space for that here. We consider only the syndrome of severe bacterial sepsis, which can be the end result of many bacterial infections in any system of the body. See Table 2.11, Figure 2.11.

The key features of infection are these: fever (although sometimes they are hypothermic), tachycardia, possibly shivering and rigors. The blood pressure can be low as the capillaries leak fluid into the extra-cellular space. There can be mental confusion. The blood tests show a high white count and CRP, a low albumin, and eventually normo-cytic normochromic anaemia.

The important result of the falling BP is renal failure. Urine output falls, and the creatinine and plasma potassium rise. The patient may become acidotic. The patients are typically hypoxic.

In severe cases, 'consumptive coagulopathy' can happen. The clotting cascades get triggered, using up clotting factors. The platelets get used up and thrombocytopenia is seen. The body runs out of stocks of unactivated clotting factor and spontaneous bleeding is seen.

The treatment for sepsis consists of antibiotics (obviously), circulatory support with fluids and adrenergic infusions such as dobutamine ('inotropic support'), oxygen, possibly dialysis to support the kidneys, and fresh frozen plasma to support coagulation. Many, many other interventions may be required, such as ventilation, and the question of 'fundamental diagnosis' is key. These patients can go bad on you very quickly.

It is striking fact that the difficulties in management of severe sepsis lie not in killing the invading bacteria but in the circulatory catastrophe that is such a major part of the septic reaction (see Useful Box 2.42). The show becomes an exercise in cardiovascular management.

Table 2.11. Major Sepsis: Summary.

Point	*Comment*
Classic features in a severe case	Fever, rigors, hypotension, tachycardia, warm peripheries ('septic shock'). Later, acidosis, poor urine output, clouding of consciousness, confusion.
To look out for	One must 'look out for' the source of the infection. The most notorious occult source is the heart valves.
Progression	Can be very rapid. When I was a registrar a 48 year-old teacher just slipped out of our hands in 24 hours. She had pneumococcal meningitis.
Terminal events	Circulatory collapse, meaning an unsupportable blood pressure which cannot be kept up by intravenous fluids or pressor drugs. Renal failure, for sure. Can end in cardiac arrest.
Likely causes	The commonest sites where serious sepsis begins are gut, followed by lung, urinary tract and skin.
Rare but treatable causes	Should all be 'treatable'... but it remains that the mortality of advanced sepsis is high, and you must be prepared for this.
Acute forms	Almost always acute!
Tests to be done	FBC, U&E, CRP, liver function, blood cultures, and other cultures (MSU, stool, sputum, CSF, joints, pus if available), imaging of suspected sites of origin of the sepsis: CXR, abdominal ultrasound or CT, lumbar puncture, cardiac echo, PET scan in some less-than-acute cases.
Treatment	Obviously antibiotics; fluids, possibly including plasma; transfusion if needed; sometimes pressor agents if the BP and the urine output are low; monitoring in ITU can be very useful; kidneys can fail, requiring some form of renal support.
Prognosis	As 'mixed' as it gets: live or die. In serious sepsis, a stage of 'multi-organ failure' can be reached (see Section 3.5) from which it is very difficult to rescue the patient, even though you have a diagnosis and have got the antibiotics started. The mortality of full-scale 'septic shock' is 50%.

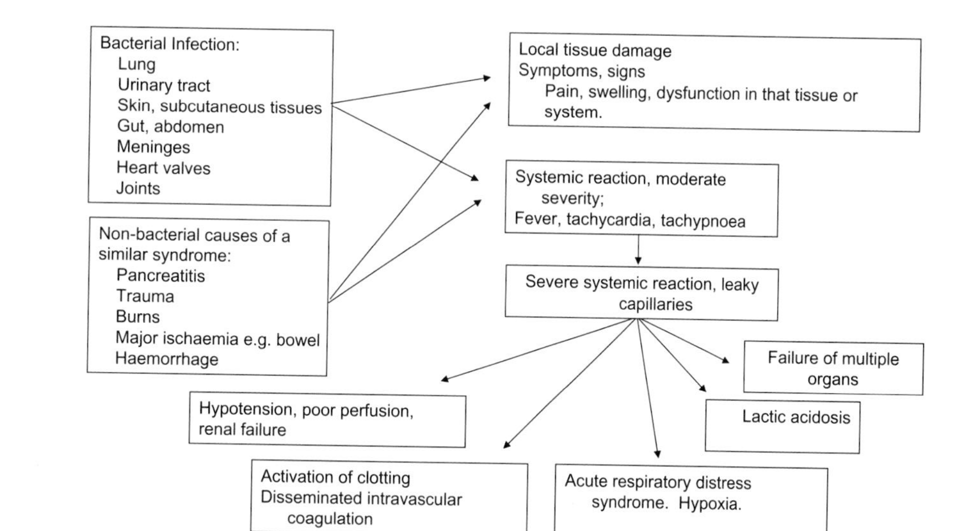

Figure 2.11. The Progression of Major Sepsis. Bacterial sepsis in any of the major systems causes a local problem in that system, and a systemic reaction which is common to all. Other major pathologies (lower left box) including trauma, burns, haemorrhage, pancreatitis can cause the same reaction. There is fever, leucocytosis, high CRP, tachycardia, hypotension. Next follows hypoperfusion, renal failure, disseminated intravascular coagulation, acute respiratory distress syndrome and failure of other organs.

Useful Box 2.41. Asplenia. The spleen can be removed without apparent immediate ill effect. The blood film looks different, and radiologists have more to write about in their reports of the abdominal CT and ultrasound, but the patient will not notice much difference... typically. The problem about the asplenic patient is that he or she is more than normally susceptible to septicaemia caused by 'encapsulated organisms' (pneumococus, haemophilus, meningococcus, group B streptococci, salmonella). Once the infection gets a hold, it can attack the asplenic patient with ferocity, taking the patient from well-being to septic shock in 24 hours or less (it's like 'neutropenic sepsis). Asplenic patients should be vaccinated against these bacteria where possible, and sometimes take daily low-dose penicillin, although this is not universal.

Useful Box 2.42. Pathophysiology of Sepsis. I think that the best way to think about 'major sepsis' is to think of the inflammatory reaction that goes with a simple skin infection, and then imagine what it would be like if the processes going on in the localised skin lesion were generally distributed around the body. So: we have the secretion of 'inflammatory mediators', those cytokine whatnots that activate inflammatory cells. The arterioles dilate up and the region becomes red and hot. The capillaries become leaky and the tissue at the site of infection swells up. The neutrophils from the blood arrive and move out from the circulation into the inflamed area. Clotting factors are activated, possibly by 'tissue factor' escaping from the interstitial fluid into the blood through the leaky capillaries. Imagine that this was happening in every blood vessel in the body. All arterioles dilate at once, and the blood pressure crashes. The capillaries become leaky and the plasma just disappears into the subcutaneous tissues. The neutrophils march out of the circulation. The clotting factors are used up.

2.12. MAJOR HAEMORRHAGE

Acute blood loss can happen for many reasons. Usually the diagnosis is clear because blood is appearing from a major wound, or is being vomited or passed as melaena. Substantial quantities of blood can be lost into internal body spaces, such as the peritoneal space (from e.g. spleen or ectopic pregnancy), or into the retroperitoneal space or into the subcutaneous tissues, in which case the helpful diagnostic sign of frank bleeding may not be present. Whatever the cause, the patient will show the following succession of symptoms and signs (see Table 2.12): light-headedness or fainting especially on standing, possibly with disturbance of vision (the retinal circulation is very sparing), tachycardia, rapid breathing, postural fall in BP, low BP lying down, weak, thready pulse, cold peripheries, diminution in urine output, clouding of consciousness. See Useful Box 2.43.

If there is no obvious bleeding, the diagnosis can be difficult. After all, there are many causes of such a clinical deterioration with low BP and a tachycardia. In sepsis, the patient should be feverish, in pulmonary embolus there should be severe cyanosis. The patient in 'cardiogenic shock' (where the myocardium has been very severely hit by infarction and cannot pump) should have signs of myocardial infarction on the ECG. Fluid loss need not be due to haemorrhage. Simple fluid deprivation, or vomiting, or diarrhoea, or uncontrolled polyuria, or loss of fluids through the skin, perhaps because of burns, can give a similar result. Acute adrenal insufficiency, a 'salt-losing' condition, can do this too, but not suddenly.

Obviously the treatment is firstly to stop the bleeding and secondly to replace the blood loss, by transfusion if possible (Useful Box 2.44), and get control of the circulation. A central venous pressure line, to measure filling of the vascular system, and a urinary catheter to measure urine output, can be very useful.

Table 2.12. Major Haemorrhage.

Point	*Comment*
Classic features in a severe case	A flat patient, sick, lying listlessly back on the trolley. Possibly pale but not necessarily. Clouding of consciousness: a bit sleepy, a bit mentally slow and perhaps drowsy. Unexpectedly cold hands and tip of the nose. A fast, weak, 'thready' pulse like the patter of a mouse. Low blood pressure that falls even further when you sit (or if possible stand) the patient up.
To look out for	The source of the bleeding can be difficult to determine. Watch the urine output; if low, keep watching the potassium and creatinine.
Progression	Rapid, can be.
Terminal events	If bleeding just cannot be stopped, cardiac arrest will happen. If BP remains low, it is the kidneys that suffer first and the patient goes into acute tubular necrosis (the pathological result of renal hypoperfusion) or at least pre-renal renal failure.
Likely causes	Trauma. GI bleeding from varices or peptic ulcer. Intraperitoneal bleeding from ectopic pregnancy (a pregnancy developing in the fallopian tube where there is no room for expansion) or ruptured spleen. Ruptured abdominal aneurysm (which is of course retroperitoneal).
Rare but treatable causes	We saw a patient once with an antibody to Factor VIII: she had an acquired form of haemophilia, in fact. The bleeding went into the subcutaneous tissues. A 'clotting screen' pointed to the diagnosis.
Acute forms	This is all acute.
Tests to be done	Pulse and blood pressure. Establish the cause (sometimes involves GI endoscopy or sometimes CT scan). Peritoneal tap if intraperitoneal bleeding is suspected. Menstrual history (if ectopic is possible). FBC, U&E, blood sample for cross matching and transfusion.
Treatment	Large bore cannulae (plural), fluids, blood, CVP line, (in ITU they would put in CVP and arterial lines), urinary catheter to monitor urine output accurately.
Prognosis	It's typically good.

Useful Box 2.43. Importance of Pulse and BP in Circulatory Assessment. The pulse and blood pressure seem so trivial to the medical student. The problem is that it is in fact very difficult to assess the circulating blood volume at the bedside. Our colleagues in ITU can use an indwelling arterial line and a dilution technique, but this is not available down in Casualty or in a general ward (in the UK). No blood test or X-ray is going to tell you the answer. The best we have is the BP. If you can get it, the 'postural fall' in BP is a useful measurement. With the patient lying on his or her back, put the cuff on and take the pressure with the patient lying supine; then keeping your stethoscope on the artery, get the patient to stand up (if he or she can, of course), and keep taking the pressure repeatedly as the patient moves to the standing position.

Useful Box 2.44. Hazards of Major Blood Transfusion. 'Major Blood Transfusion' means something like more than 10 units in 24 hours. It has its risks. Transmission of an infection, such as a virus, becomes possible. The protein content of the plasma will not be optimal: coagulopathy is the overt result here. Transfused red cells are not the best oxygen carriers. No useful platelets will be transfused; the risk of an allergic reaction to red or white cells or platelets increases.

2.13. CANCER

'Cancer' is a huge topic. It affects every system. There are two main types; 'solid' tumours such as lung, breast, gut, prostate, and the 'soft' tumours of the haematological system, leukaemias and lymphomas.

As you know, the fundamental pathology is a molecular mistake that gives rise to a clone of cells with uncontrolled proliferation. It is reckoned that there is a 24 month lead-in time before the swelling becomes detectable by even the most sensitive of imaging techniques. Growth is exponential.

The solid tumours are commoner. They go through at least two stages; confined, and metastatic in which the tumour spreads via the bloodstream or lymphatics to distant sites.

Diagnosis has two phases. It is first very important to get a 'histological diagnosis' by the biopsy of the abnormal tissue. Then there is are scans aimed at 'staging', finding out how far it has spread.

There are many ways of assessing spread and severity. CT scanning is perhaps the most commonly-used. MRI is not far behind. PET-scanning (positron emission tomography) searches for tissues that have a high metabolic rate. The patient is injected with a modified glucose molecule labelled with the isotope ^{18}fluorine. If the tissue is actively metabolising (could be cancerous, might be infective) then it shows up as 'hot'. Some tumours are associated with abnormalities detectable in the blood, so-called 'tumour markers', of which 'prostate-specific antigen' or PSA is perhaps the best known; this is an easily-measurable blood level for prostate cancer.

After staging, comes treatment. If the tumour is single and is surgically accessible, then hopefully it can be removed. If not, then radiotherapy and/or chemotherapy may be available (which bring their own problems of haematological and/or immune failure). The haematological malignancies, leukaemia and lymphoma, will not be cured by surgery and so treatment goes direct to chemotherapy and possibly bone marrow transplantation if there is a suitable donor.

Cancer patients can present with a huge array of clinical problems, in any system of the body. The primary tumour can cause pressure problems, wherever it might be, blocking a tube in the lung or the gut or a kidney. Tumours, which have a rough-and-ready blood supply, tend to bleed, causing haemoptysis, haematuria or GI blood loss. Pain due to expansion is possible. It is the secondary spread that usually causes the more serious problems, as multiple target organs are infiltrated with growing secondary tumours. Favourite target organs depend on the primary, but can be liver, bone, lung, lymph gland or brain.

There are a series of classical oncological emergencies that can occur; spinal cord compression by tumour in a vertebral body, superior vena caval obstruction by a mediastinal tumour, airway obstruction in the lung leading to stridor, severe hypercalcaemia (caused by destruction of bone) and raised intracranial pressure from brain metastases. Under treatment, massive lysis of tumour cells can lead to a surge in the plasma level of uric acid, which is a renal toxin and can cause gout. The treatment of cancer with chemotherapy often leads to immune suppression in many forms, often neutropenia.

'Cachexia' is a common cancer-related problem, but can also occur in many other contexts, such as cardiac failure, AIDS, other chronic infections, gut failure. It is a weight-losing state, with loss of not only fat but also muscle. The muscle wasting causes weakness and debility; it can be seen as a concavity over the temples, where the temporalis muscles have wasted. It is associated with a loss of appetite, susceptibility to infection and is notoriously hard to treat.

It is the case that many patients in oncology die of the disease. The oncologist plays a large part in palliative care.

2.14. SOME WORDS ABOUT BLOOD GASES

The arterial blood gas is a key investigation in many conditions. It gives vital information on the physiology relating gas content and acid-base balance. Acid base and respiratory gases are tightly-linked in many ways. Carbon dioxide converts to an acid: more CO_2, more acid, acidosis; less CO_2, less acid, alkalosis. In addition to acidosis/alkalosis caused by respiratory changes in CO_2, if there is a primary disorder of acid balance (e.g. the alkalosis of vomiting) the body counters the metabolic 'pressure' by varying the ventilation rate to vary the pCO_2: in metabolic acidosis, the body hyperventilates to induce a compensatory respiratory alkalosis; in metabolic alkalosis, there is a degree of hypoventilation to induce a compensatory respiratory acidosis. See Tables 2.13 and 2.14.

Many very sick patients are acidotic. There are many reasons. The lungs may not be working well for a start, reducing both oxygen supply and carbon dioxide excretion. The low oxygen tension is transmitted to the tissues and they are pushed into a degree of anaerobic metabolism, which yields lactate, an organic acid, giving a metabolic acidosis. If the kidneys are failing, a main route of acid excretion is blocked, further exacerbating the metabolic acidosis. As you can imagine a patient like this could easily have a mixed respiratory and metabolic acidosis.

There is a link between acid-base balance and the concentration of potassium in the plasma. It is often (but not always) the case that acidosis is associated with hyperkalaemia, and alkalosis with hypokalaemia. When the acid-base problem is corrected the potassium comes back to normal. This is best seen in the treatment of diabetic ketoacidosis. The patient comes in with a potassium of something like 5.5 mmol/l, which begins to drop quickly when the acidosis comes under control.

For words on 'anion gap' and 'osmotic gap', see Useful Box 2.45.

Table 2.13. System Failures. Summary: Arterial Blood Gases. Normal values: pO_2, 10–13 kPa; pCO_2, 4.8–6.1 kPa; pH, 7.35–7.45; HCO_3, 22–26 mmol/l.

Description	*Typical numbers*	*Bicarbonate*	*Clinical state*	*To think about*	*Comment*
Metabolic acidosis	pO_2, 15 pCO_2, 4 pH, 7.1 HCO_3 8	Down to 3 sometimes	Very often 'ill' because of the typically serious fundamental pathology. Possibly hyperventilating.	Methanol or antifreeze (ethylene glycol) poisonings: high anion and osmotic gaps.	The simplest is diabetic ketoacidosis, due to aceto-acetic and beta hydroxybutyric acids. Lactic acidosis comes next.
Respiratory acidosis	pO_2, 6 pCO_2, 12 pH 7.1 HCO_3 32	High	Cyanosed, drowsy, jerking: a carbon-dioxide-retention 'flap'.	Neurology: depression of respiration by opiates; muscle weakness e.g. myasthenia.	Often the final event in respiratory failure.
Metabolic alkalosis	pO_2, 9 pCO_2, 8 pH 7.55 HCO_3 34	High	First symptom is paraesthesiae. The muscles then begin to tighten, into 'tetany'.	Often the result of vomiting. Diuretics cause a degree of metabolic alkalosis.	Both alkaloses, respiratory and metabolic, can show 'tetany': spontaneously active sensory and motor peripheral nerves.
Respiratory alkalosis	pO_2, 14 pCO_2, 3.5 pH 7.52 HCO_3 16	Low	Ditto	Often the result of some form of hyperventilation. Can be psychological in origin. Salicylate overdose can cause hyperventilation.	The least problematic of the blood gas abnormalities.

Table 2.14. Individual Measurements in the ABG. Let's consider the individual measurements one by one.

Measurement	*Comment*
pO_2	A low pO_2 is the commonest abnormality, signifying poor gas exchange, due to either a lung problem (which may be fundamentally cardiac) or decreased breathing effort.
pCO_2	pCO_2 can often either be raised or lowered. CO_2 acts like an acid while oxygen is neither acidic nor basic. So in addition to changes in pCO_2 due to gas exchange abnormalities, the body can often manipulate pCO_2 to vary the pH. The classic example is metabolic acidosis, where compensatory hyperventilation drives the pCO_2 down and the pH up.
pH	A very fundamental blood measurement. Correct pH is vital for the function of all proteins and for proper membrane excitability. Alkalosis gives neurological hyperexcitability, manifest as paraesthesiae and tetany. The clinical picture of acidosis is dominated by hyperventilation, the compensatory respiratory reaction.
Bicarbonate	Goes up when pCO_2 goes up, and down when pCO_2 goes down. A useful independent measure of acid-base status. The *venous* bicarbonate is a very useful measurement of blood gas status.
Lactate	A useful measure almost always pointing to something serious if it is abnormally high. High after cardiac arrest and after an authentic grand mal seizure; high in severe sepsis and in some major infarctive conditions where much tissue becomes gangrenous, especially in gut infarction.

Useful Box 2.45. Anion and Osmotic Gaps. We should look at two related quantities that can also matter very much, if not very often, one night many years from now when you are in Casualty.

Anion gap	The difference between the 'measured cations' and the 'measured anions'. If it is high then the gap has to be filled by an organic anion e.g. lactate or acetoacetic/betahydroxybutyrate (in DKA) or some other anion, e.g. salicylate.
Osmotic gap	The difference between the measured osmolarity and the measurable constituents contributing to the plasma osmolarity. If increased, there is an abnormal osmolyte lurking about, typically methanol or ethylene glycol.

3

Some Typical Patient Pictures

In the next pages we will consider some of the classic types of patients that are encountered in a UK hospital. You will see how the system failures and dysfunctions keep coming up in the different patient types.

Like all medical textbooks, this one gives idealised generalizations of clinical medicine. The reality on the wards is often less clear, quite messy and indefinite. But we have to start out in medicine with the kind of generalization described here. As time goes by you will see a lot of bizarre situations, which can temporarily bias your perception of what makes up 'common' medicine. As you get more and more experience under your belt you will appreciate how patients tend to fall into groups which makes diagnosis easier. A few of these 'patient pictures' are given here in this chapter.

We consider the arteriopath, the alcoholic, the psychotic, the IVDU, the very sick patient, the elderly patient and the very obese. Each type comes with a characteristic series of possible problems that one should be thinking about as one assesses the patient type.

These patient pictures are useful because they have diagnostic value. One of my former students proudly proclaimed, 'Prof Stewart taught me how to stereotype'. Well, it's true, I admit it, I did. In modern parlance, the word 'stereotype' is pejorative, but the fact is that patients follow patterns and these are useful to understand. Your main job is to make the correct diagnosis, and the quicker you can do that, the better. You start by guessing (er, 'hypothesising') and then you narrow the possibilities as you move forward through the history and the tests. The cute thing to do is to guess well in the early stages, so that you can choose the right tests and get to the correct answer quickly. We may not actually do the algebra, but in our reasoning we say to ourselves, 'We've got this symptom, in this patient, with this background. What are the likelihoods of these diagnoses?' We mentally exercise what is understood in mathematics as 'Bayesian probability'. We modify the probability of a particular diagnosis in the light of the situation in front of us.

The patient might have chest pain. A common diagnosis might be coronary artery disease. If the patient is 68, a smoker and has already been admitted six times with chest pain, and previous tests including a coronary angiogram have been abnormal, then coronary artery disease is indeed very likely. If the patient is age 8, and has recently had a violent squabble with his big brother, then coronary artery disease is unlikely. Note that I didn't say that it's actually 'impossible' (because he might just have a congenital abnormality of his coronary arteries), just 'unlikely'. An ECG is unlikely to be a helpful test, and you will think very long and very hard about an invasive and potentially risky coronary angiogram.

So this kind of 'stereotyping' is about *probability*, not *certainty*. It's about what to look for first, so that you can get to the right answer quickly. If your tests are negative (and your original hypothesis is therefore probably wrong), so be it. and you have to look again, but at least you have followed a sensible path.

3.1. THE ARTERIOPATH

The arteriopath (Table 3.1, Figure 3.1) is a very common patient in British medicine. Usually a smoker, more commonly male, he or she has widespread atheromatous disease. Perhaps the most likely arteries to be affected are the coronaries, closely followed by the carotids and the iliacs/femorals. The mesenterics and renals do not escape. Narrowing of the coronaries gives three major clinical conditions: angina (central chest pain on exercise relieved by rest), myocardial infarction (complete blockage resulting in some muscle loss) and cardiac failure, Section 2.1. Narrowing of the carotids gives TIAs and full-scale stroke. Narrowing of the iliacs/femorals gives intermittent claudication or worse, an ischaemic limb (Useful Box 3.1). Narrowing of the renal arteries gives silent renal failure. Narrowing of mesenteric vessels can give abdominal pain on eating, or if the blockage is complete, the urgent surgical emergency of mesenteric infarction with gangrenous bowel.

Investigation in many systems is by Doppler ultrasound or angiogram, least invasively performed by MRI. The ECG is very helpful for coronary disease; CT and MRI in the brain. Treatment is largely in the domain of the interventional radiologist and surgeon. Apart from the thrombolytic 'clot buster' enzymes (Useful Box 3.2), drug treatment does not help much. Statins and aspirin are largely preventive.

Atheroma is not the only arterial disease out there, but it is by far the commonest. There are the inflammatory 'vasculitis' conditions, typically affecting small arteries and not associated with the blockage of large arteries. Some inflammatory conditions of the arteries (temporal arteritis, Takayusu's, polyarteritis nodosa) do affect the larger vessels.

Aside from 'simple' atheroma, diabetes is the main medical condition affecting arterial blood supply, and is of course often seen in the same patients who have atheroma.

Table 3.1. The Arteriopath: Summary.

Point	*Comment*
Classic features in a severe case	Smoker of 70 with claudication, angina and something of a stroke history; either TIAs or a full blown hemiplegia. Will typically have a degree of COPD as well. Possibly 'intermittent claudication'. Physical examination reveals absent, reduced or delayed peripheral pulses, with bruits most easily audible at femorals and carotids, possibly at subclavians and in the abdomen. Coronary disease is also likely. Abnormal neurology.
To look out for	The kidneys can suffer as well of course, but the pathology is rarely diagnosed, although MRI does help. Aneurysms (see Useful Box 3.1).
Progression	Over years, stutteringly; meaning with sudden exacerbations.
Terminal events	Stroke, cardiac ischaemia, infection of ischaemic limb. Occasionally gut ischaemia, or renal ischaemia.
Likely causes	Smoking, diabetes.
Rare but treatable causes	Takayusu's disease occurs in young ladies of Far Eastern origin. Temporal arteritis and polyarteritis nodosa are steroid-suppressible diseases that affect larger arteries.
Acute forms	Many acute presentations here.
Remember	Intravenous X-ray contrast medium can be nephrotoxic.
Tests to be done	ECG, CXR, U&E, FBC, ESR, cholesterol, Doppler studies, angiograms, by X-ray or by MRI.
Treatment	Vasodilators? Not much use. Stop smoking (that's a laugh). Surgery or interventional radiology: carotid endarterectomy; femoro-popliteal bypass, coronary stents. Statins are useful for prevention.
Prognosis	Unpredictable

Useful Box 3.1. How to Feel the Popliteal Pulses. Flex the patient's knee to 90°. Put your two thumbs on the patient's tibial tuberosity anteriorly. Sink your middle fingers into the popliteal fossa at the back and try to catch the popliteal artery between your fingertips and the posterior aspect of the tibia.

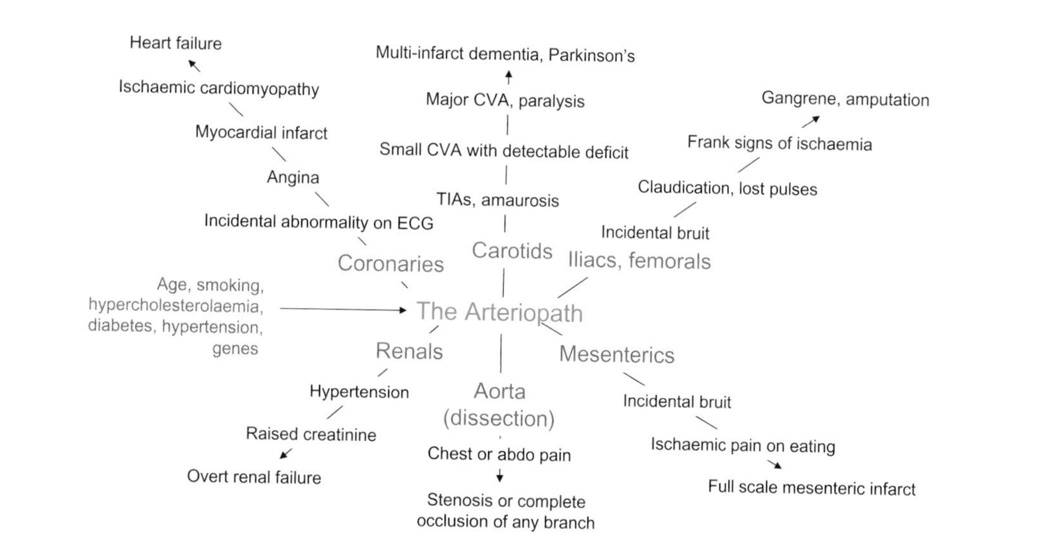

Figure 3.1. Map: The Arteriopath. It is the nature of the patchy arteriosclerotic disease that one set of arteries is going to give problems before any other, but physical examination or investigations in the patient often show problems in the other major arteries. As usual, the kidneys and its arteries are the hardest to know about, the silent sufferers that they are. Magnetic resonance arteriography is very useful here. ('Aortic dissection' in this diagram: see Useful Box 3.3.)

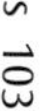

Useful Box 3.2. Thrombolytic Treatment for Acute Infarction. 'Clot busters' have been in regular use for myocardial infarction for many years and have made a big difference to outcomes. Stroke has been more difficult to treat this way, since haemorrhagic stroke can happen and if this is the diagnosis, clot busters will make things worse. It is now becoming conventional to give TPA (tissue plasminogen activator) within 3 hours of the onset of the event if a CT has ruled out haemorrhage and if there are no contraindications e.g. severe hypertension or recent bleeding event.

Useful Box 3.3. 'Aneurysm' is a potential problem in the arteriopath. In its original meaning, taken from the Greek 'aneurysma', it meant a widening. The modern meaning certainly includes abnormal widening of blood vessels, but the word is also used to describe 'dissecting' pathology of the aortic wall in which the aorta need not necessarily be enlarged, although it usually is. In dissection, the main abnormality is that there arises a hole in the intima, admitting the blood under pressure to the media, tearing the intima away from the adventitia and thus creating a new conduit for the blood. Although such a vessel can undoubtedly increase in overall diameter, it need not do. The unifying feature in 'aneurysm' is weakness or tearing of the structure of the wall of the vessel, and this is (I think) how the word is used now.

In a straightforward aneurysm, such as one might see in the abdominal aorta or circle of Willis, there is a simple bulge. I am not going to go on about it now, but 'Laplace's Law' in physics means that as the wall of the vessel stretches and gets bigger, it has to work even harder to contain the blood under pressure within the aneurysm. But the aortic wall has stretched and become thinner and therefore weaker, so the situation is an unstable one and rupture is a distinct possibility.

Whatever the nature of the aneurysm, possible outcomes can include rupture, thrombosis, embolism and occlusion of the origins of branches. In aneurysms of the ascending aorta, the mountings for the aortic valve can stretch, causing the valve to leak. We saw such a case today.

3.2. THE ALCOHOLIC

The alcoholic is a very common visitor to the British hospital, and has been for a very long time. William Hogarth's famous London etching 'Gin Lane' depicts massive alcohol problems in 1751. In 2010, the young acutely intoxicated is a short-term casualty problem. It is those who have been drinking for decades that become very severely ill. There are about six major problems for the chronic alcoholic (see Table 3.2 and Figure 3.2). Liver disease ending in cirrhosis with decompensated liver failure, is the single commonest fate (Section 2.4). Ethanol is toxic to the pancreas, giving pancreatitis with eventual failure of both exocrine and endocrine aspects of the organ. Ethanol is toxic to the heart, giving the condition 'alcoholic cardiomyopathy', a cause of cardiac failure (Section 2.1). Ethanol is a neurotoxin: the cerebellum and peripheral nerves are the earliest victims of its toxicity in the nervous system (Sections 2.7.2.4 and 2.7.2.7). Alcoholics often present with seizures. The other problem of the alcoholic is the social slide into destitution that accompanies alcohol addiction.

The inebriated alcoholic comes to Casualty. Your tasks are these. Somehow or another you have to obtain some kind of history and examine the patient. You will have to deal with the major presenting problem (e.g. GI bleed). Your assessments will include physical examination and blood tests and X-rays looking at the heart, liver, gut and neurological function. It is routine to start benzodiazepine 'cover' to prevent the acute organic psychosis 'delirium tremens' (see Useful Box 3.5). It is also routine to give a vitamin combo ('Pabrinex') containing thiamine to prevent Wernicke's encephalopathy (see Useful Box 3.6).

Scabies (Useful Box 3.7) is common in the homeless. Alcoholism is often associated with dependence on other chemicals (Useful Box 3.8).

During all this you have to keep your eyes open. One time in 50, such a patient will be harbouring another clinical problem that is not immediately evident in the initial assessment. Subdural haematoma is the classic, but there are many others.

Table 3.2. The Alcoholic.

Point	*Comment*
Classic features in a severe case	Chronic liver disease (see 'Liver Failure', Section 2.4) is obviously the most common presentation of chronic heavy alcohol use, but let us not forget pancreatic disease and failure (malabsorption, diabetes: Useful Box 3.4), cerebellar failure (Section 2.7.2.4), peripheral neuropathy (Section 2.7.2.7), epilepsy, and cardiomyopathy with heart failure (Section 2.1). The alcoholic also typically has social problems: joblessness, poverty, family break up, isolation; a vicious cycle develops in which the patient drinks even more alcohol to escape the unpleasantness of this isolation.
To look out for	It is a notorious Casualty thing that the 'drunk' is sometimes harbouring an underlying diagnosis that is masked by the intoxication. One patient that we had at UCH had a C5 spinal cord contusion (well done, Dr J).
Progression	Typically over years.
Terminal events	Typically, in terminal liver failure, but there are many other outcomes.
Likely causes	Not applicable.
Rare but treatable causes	Do not mistake the cerebellar ataxic (Section 2.7.2.4) for an alcoholic.
Acute forms	Delirium tremens, variceal bleed, seizures, acute pancreatitis, heart failure, atrial fibrillation.
Tests to be done	FBC including MCV, U&E, LFT, PTT, ultrasound of liver and abdomen, CXR, ECG, amylase, often CT head, possibly EEG.
Treatment	Must cover possibilities of Wernicke's and DTs with vitamin B complex and benzodiazepines respectively. Management of the alcohol addiction is difficult. See 'liver failure' for hepatic problems.
Prognosis	Not good unless the patient can resist the temptation, which is hard.

Useful Box 3.4. Jeffrey Bernard was a journalist on *The Spectator* whose extremely entertaining weekly 'Low Life' column charted his gradual alcoholic decline. It was pancreatitis that he developed, making him diabetic, giving him arterial problems (and an amputation) and then renal failure. He started on dialysis but could not tolerate the restrictions on his fluid intake, and baled out in December 1997. Five days later, he died. It was presumably a hyperkalaemic death, so it was hopefully painless and peaceful.

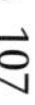

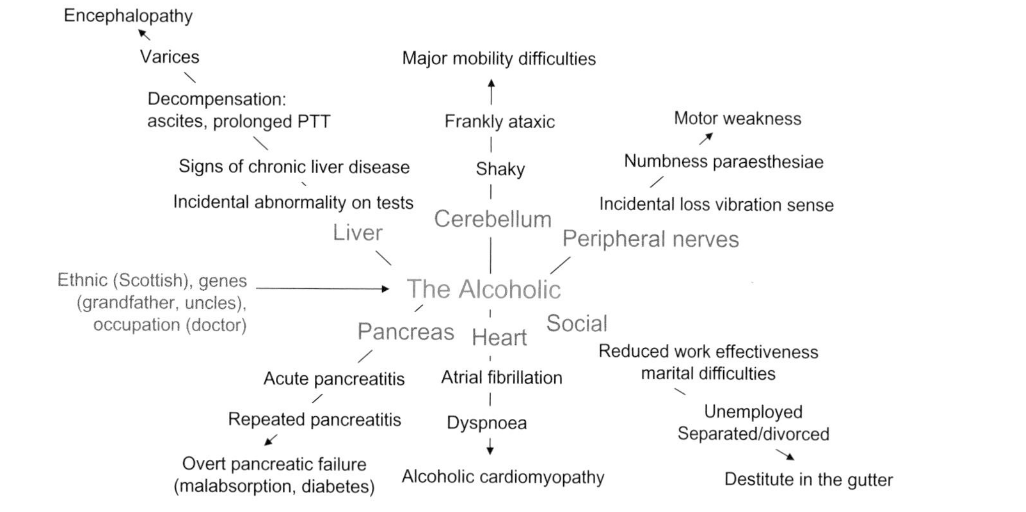

Figure 3.2. Map: The Alcoholic. It is not just liver disease from which alcoholics come to suffer. Alcohol is toxic to the nervous system, especially the cerebellum and peripheral nerves; to the heart, where it causes atrial fibrillation and heart failure; and to the pancreas, where it causes acute and chronic pancreatitis. The alcoholic also suffers social problems, often losing spouse, job, family contacts, house and income.

Useful Box 3.5. Delirium Tremens (DTs) is the 'acute organic psychosis' ('organic' because it has a chemical or anatomical cause; 'psychosis', a brain malfunction characterised by loss of contact with reality) associated with sudden withdrawal of alcohol from the dependent. It is a real risk of hospital admission. There is a progression: the patient is admitted and has his or her presenting problems sorted out. After 12 hours he or she becomes shaky and feels nervous. After 24 hours he or she is sweaty, even shakier, and getting agitated. At 36 hours he or she suddenly goes berserk, beset by tremendously frightening visual hallucinations which make him or her very upset. On one occasion the hallucinating DTs patient accused me of being a 'bodkin' (which is apparently a kind of dagger). 'You're a bodkin! You're a bodkin!' he screamed at the top of his voice, in terror. Looking back, this should never have happened. We knew he was a drinker and we should have had him covered from admission, and we should have spotted the agitation-tremor-sweating signs before he got to the hallucinating stage, and given him the benzos. Osler: 'Experience is the sum of your mistakes'.

Useful Box 3.6. Wernicke's Encephalopathy. Wernicke was a German neurologist whose first name I forget now. He died after a cycling accident. His encephalopathy is a syndrome of external ophthalmoplegia, ataxia and confusion with memory loss, all caused by deficiency of thiamine. Untreated, it can lead to Korsakoff psychosis, in which the patient is unable to store new memories after the primary insult, a most disabling problem. It is so important because it is so easily treated, with thiamine. This is why you will see so much Pabrinex given in Casualty. (NB do not confuse with 'Parvolex', which is n-acetyl cysteine given for paracetamol overdose.) Wernicke's encephalopathy is not confined to alcoholics: it is beginning to occur with reasonable frequency in patients who have recently had bariatric surgery (Section 3.7).

Useful Box 3.7. Scabies is skin disease in which an invertebrate burrows into the skin, causing intense itch and multiplies. It is often found in the 'crevasses': the skin folds, e.g. between the fingers and other more intimate places. It goes with being chronically unwashed. The skin is reddened and itchy, often scratched, and often secondarily infected with 'impetigo'-like crusting lesions. Diagnosis is not easy, and you need a dermatologist, and treatment is not simple either. But it's contagious (to other family members and to you) so it's a very useful diagnosis to make.

Useful Box 3.8. The Idea of the 'Chemically Dependent'. You will find that individuals who abuse one kind of euphoriant very often abuse others. In the realm of legal, tax-gathering chemicals, alcohol and tobacco frequently go together. But the idea extends to other substances as well: ecstasy, opiates, cannabis. Many patients just take what they can get on a particular day.

3.3. THE MEDICAL PROBLEMS OF THE PSYCHOTIC

'Psychosis' is a term for mentally ill patients who have lost contact with reality. A psychosis can be 'organic', having a basis in internal medicine, e.g. the confusion of severe fever, or it can be 'functional', what you and I would consider as 'psychiatric'. The two main functional psychoses are schizophrenia and bitemporal disorder (i.e. manic depression). Schizophrenic patients are withdrawn, eccentric people who sometimes hear voices that tell them to do some really bad things. Bipolar patients oscillate in mood, veering between mania — when they think they can fly, and depression — when they are suicidal.

The management of psychotic patients is largely in the hands of psychiatrists, but we see many psychotic patients in medical wards.

Figure 3.3 shows the many medical problems that the psychotically-ill patient can present with. The mentally-ill patient often indulges in different drugs, often opiates: these have their own side effects. The mentally-ill patient is rarely a regular attender at routine out-patient clinics: it can be difficult to manage effectively both the mental illness and any concomitant physical illnesses which might be present, such as diabetes or hypertension. The drugs prescribed for the mental illness have their own side-effects. Lithium (often used for bipolar disease) causes renal problems, while phenothiazines cause basal ganglia problems. Mental illness can give depression or delusion which can lead to overdose, often with the drugs used to treat the psychosis. The social isolation and deprivation of mental illness lead to the individual being financially destitute and to be condemned to squalid unhygienic housing, with skin infections, malnutrition and TB as possible medical complications.

It is a tragedy of our time that we do not look after these unfortunate people better.

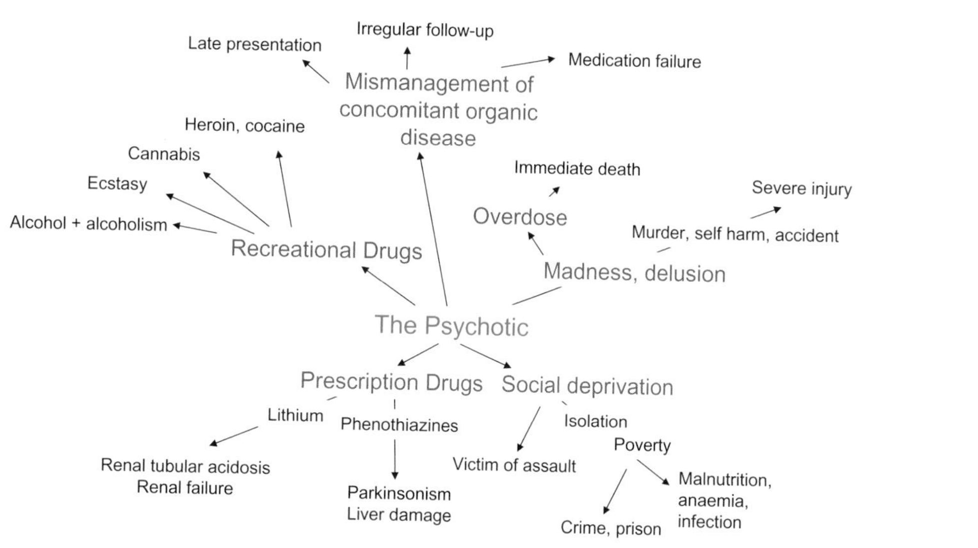

Figure 3.3. The Medical Problems of the Psychotic Patient. As if schizophrenia or bipolar disease were not hard enough, psychotic patients have more than their fair share of medical problems. They tend to abuse 'recreational' drugs, with the attendant problems there. They are not good attenders at medical clinics, so if they do have some kind of 'organic disease' the management tends to be patchy. In serious bouts of psychosis they can be subject to suicidal overdose, or to physical injury. They are not stable members of society, so they do not have regular income or housing and can get into severe deprivation. Finally the prescribed drugs are powerful and have major side-effects.

3.4. THE INTRAVENOUS DRUG USER (IVDU)

The IVDU is a common visitor to British hospitals. His or her different problems are summarised in Figure 3.4. The principal problem that he or she presents with on a medical ward is bacterial infection; at a site of injection (typically the groin or skin), or in a joint or bone by virtue of haematogenous spread, or on a heart valve in 'bacterial endocarditis'. Typically the IVDU has the worst of social circumstances. Not able to hold down a job, with a financially very demanding drug habit that often mandates regular theft to support it. The IVDU is usually beyond the law and unwilling to cooperate with what we would regard as satisfactory medical follow up.

Often, in-patient medicine is confined to damage limitation, the giving of large doses of broad spectrum antibiotics and other treatments, before the patient decides that he or she is sufficiently well to return to the streets and a ready supply of euphoric chemistry.

The main injected drug of abuse is heroin. Cocaine can be injected but is more often inhaled. Heroin is highly addictive, and the urge to obtain another dose drives the addict to extreme lengths (including murder) to get more. Acute heroin overdose leads to small pupils ('miosis'), respiratory depression with slow, shallow respiration and low oxygen saturations, bradycardia and coma. It can be treated with IV naloxone, but you must remember that the half life of naloxone is much shorter than that of heroin, so it wears off. The patient falls back into his or her hypoventilating stupor when you are off seeing to your next patient.

The world badly needs a drug that can interrupt the addictive cycle. Methadone is really just a long-acting opiate, equally addictive and orally administered. It's 'harm reduction' (no bad thing, of course) rather than cure.

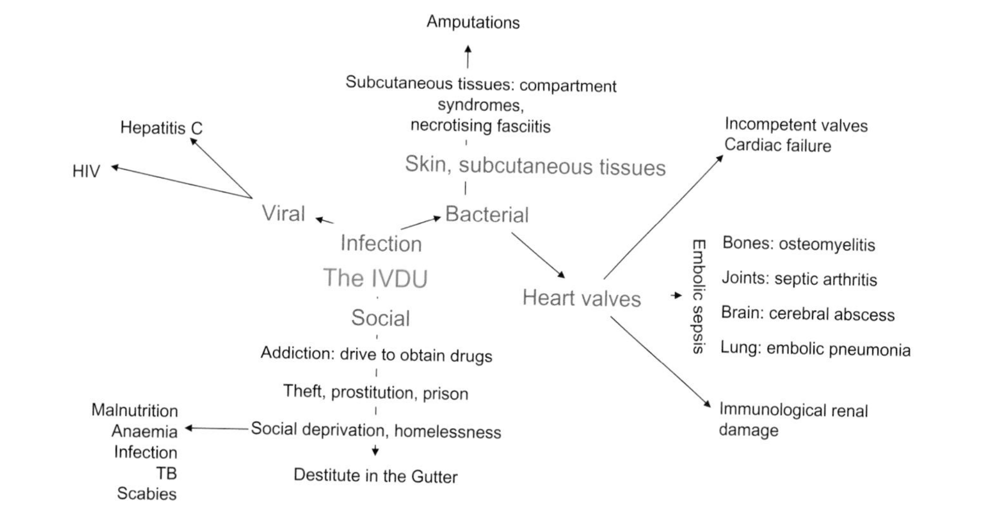

Figure 3.4. The Intravenous Drug User (IVDU). The constant injection of non-sterile impure chemicals into the veins introduces infection and thrombosis. There can be local infection in the groin and deep venous thrombosis in the femoral vein. The infection can spread via the blood; favourite destinations being the joints and the bones, occasionally the heart valves. If the infection does lodge on the valve leaflets (which have no capillary circulation) the body has no effective answer.

3.5. THE VERY SICK PATIENT

The ‘very sick patient’ is one who is at immediate risk of death. The underlying condition may be in any system and may be of any fundamental pathology. He or she will typically be following at least two of the failure syndromes described in the earlier pages of this book, a situation known as ‘multi-organ failure’, sometimes ‘multiple organ dysfunction syndrome’ (MODS). The patient may well be septic (Section 2.11), or have severe haemorrhage, acute pancreatitis, major trauma or burns, or pre-eclampsia (a hypertensive-nephrotic condition suffered by pregnant women.)

The diagram, Figure 3.5, which is really a synthesis of many of the previous failure syndrome diagrams, shows how the systems can progressively fail as the condition of the patient deteriorates.

The first systems to show dysfunction are cardiovascular (low BP, tachycardia), renal (low urine output or ‘oliguria’) and lung (leaky capillaries, oedematous lungs: ARDS).

It is inevitable that the liver tests will be abnormal. The enzymes will be raised and there is a risk of ischaemic liver damage due to poor perfusion. Leakage of tissue factor from tissues into the blood is a possible mechanism behind the activation of the clotting cascades, giving ‘disseminated intravascular coagulation’. The CNS dysfunction is mainly cognitive and brainstem in nature, but strokes can easily happen.

These patients very often (should always?) end up in intensive care. An ITU offers a level of monitoring (CVP, arterial pressure) and nursing that is not available on a general ward. The ITU can also offer artificial ventilation and haemofiltration. Their access to monitoring data allows the doctors to see physiological data (e.g. cardiac output) which we can only guess at on a general ward.

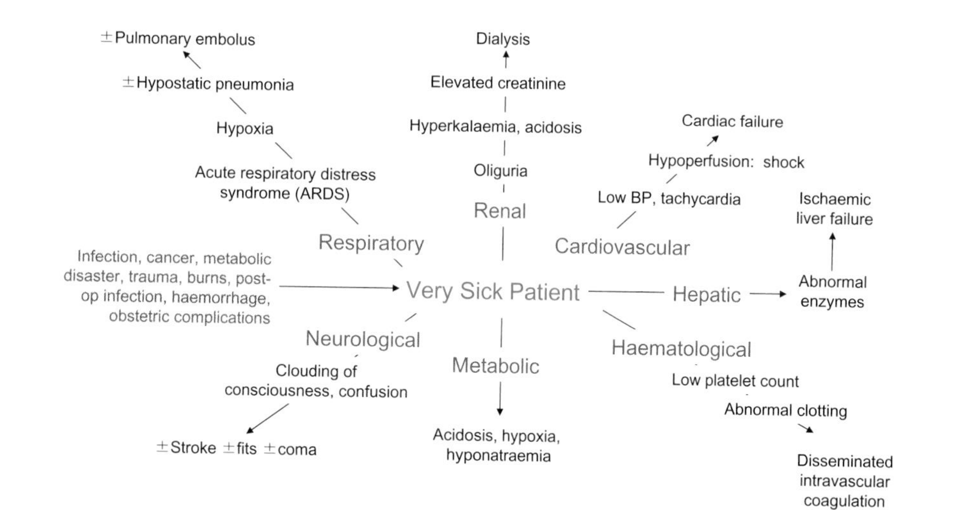

Figure 3.5. The Very Sick Patient. This map shows some of the common pathways taken in the 'very sick patient'. The patient might be septic, or have undergone very major surgery (aneurysm repair,) or have suffered serious burns. Whatever the cause, two things will probably be true: the CRP will be high, and the BP will be low. The capillaries will get leaky and will ooze plasma. The kidneys will falter: urine output will fall. The lungs will get wet (acute respiratory distress syndrome, ARDS). Metabolism does not work well in these bad circumstances, and the patient becomes acidotic. More systems start to go down. Disseminated intravascular coagulation can occur.

3.6. THE ELDERLY PATIENT

Over the age of about 80 or 85, a frailty develops in the human frame that is associated with some characteristic medical changes (see Figure 3.6). There is an accumulation of damage due to multiple past events which leave scars or other irreversible results: small infarcts in every system, scars secondary to previous infections, deposition of proteins especially in neurones, calcifications — especially in blood vessels. The striated muscles, voluntary and cardiac, weaken (this may be due to shortage of mitochondria). Heart failure can easily occur. Even if the patient is not a smoker, the lungs will have taken their share of punishment. The skin becomes thin and delicate, and will bruise easily; the gut is prone to ischaemic changes. Constipation and volvulus (a twisting of the gut on its mesentery) are common. The joints become stiff and often painful. The eyes develop cataracts and macular degeneration. The hearing and balance fail, and there is an attrition in renal tubules and therefore creatinine clearance falls. In the females there is a major susceptibility to urinary infection. The brain may have been damaged by repeated strokes, large or small, or by protein accumulation of one kind or another. The memory may be impaired and there can be a change in the personality, with loss of confidence and of volition, and sometimes paranoia. They tend to lose weight. Continence can be a problem. Useful Box 3.9 summarises some common diagnoses in the elderly.

Histories can be difficult to obtain and can be complex. Physical examination has to be interpreted in the light of the patient's age. For instance, the ankle jerks are often absent and vibration sense is often missing in the feet.

Nevertheless it can be a very satisfying professional experience, diagnosing and effectively treating conditions arising within this complex background, using practical, humane common sense to decide on the extent of intervention.

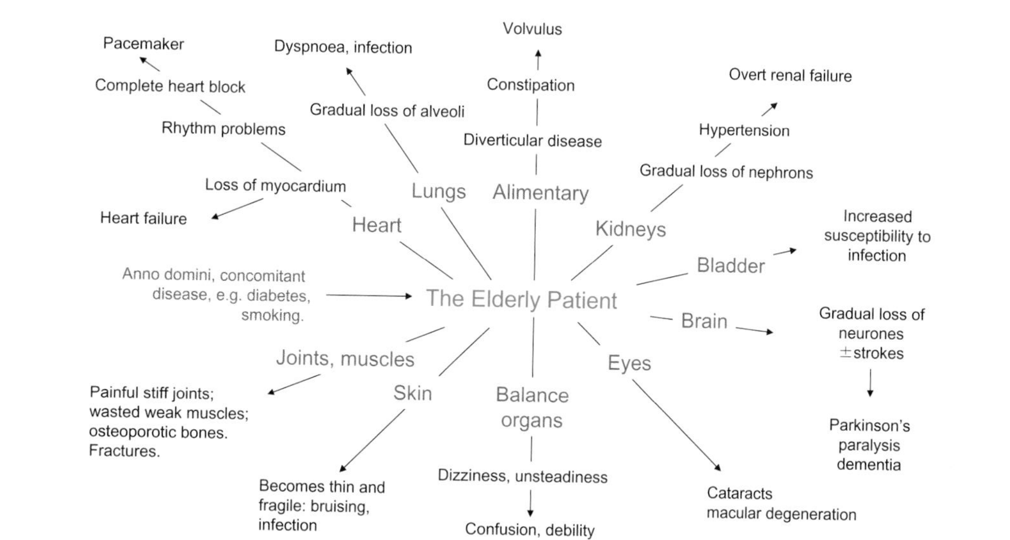

Figure 3.6. The Elderly Patient. After about 85, there is a creeping loss of functioning tissue. Some is due to the build-up of protein (e.g. Lewy bodies), or death of cells that are never replaced. There are scarred tissues, perhaps previously infarcted, loss of irreplaceable neurones, nephrons, myocardial cells, worn out joints, failing sight. The problems are not in themselves insurmountable, but it's the sum of the problems that make life so difficult. Treatment has to be practical and simple and not have too many side effects. There is a lot of occupational therapy/physiotherapy/social worker support to be put in.

Useful Box 3.9. Common Conditions in the Elderly. It is all too easy to dismiss vague symptoms in the elderly as being simply due to 'the patient's age'. It is better for the patient, and more satisfying for you, to make a real diagnosis. We have mentioned many of the common conditions of the elderly (cardiac failure, coronary artery disease, chronic obstructive airways disease, hypothyroidism, diabetes, stroke, Alzheimer's, osteoarthritis) but here are some other problems that keep on cropping up.

AV Conducting System Dysfunction. Rhythm problems are common in the elderly and can give blackouts and/or cardiac failure. Atrial fibrillation needs to have its 'default' rapid rate controlled. Heart block (and many variants) often require a pacemaker.

The dyspnoea of **pleural effusion** creeps up on the patient gradually, usually without pain or cough or wheeze. It should be easy to diagnose clinically, with stony dullness and absent breath sounds at the base on the affected side.

Cataract is visible via the ophthalmoscope and is relatively easy to treat surgically, under local anaesthetic.

Electrolyte Problems are common. Hyponatraemia is seen in cardiac and liver failures, and can be caused by diuretics. Very occasionally it is caused by ADH secretion from a lung tumour. Hypernatraemia is seen in the summer in residents of care homes, when the evaporative fluid loss exceeds intake. Hypokalaemia is most commonly caused by diuretics but diarrhoea and/or vomiting are good causes. Hyperkalaemia occurs in renal failure, after treatment with spironolactone and sometimes in diabetics.

Pernicious Anaemia is a most satisfying thing to diagnose and treat. Gradually increasing fatigue; low Hb (perhaps 4–5 g/dl) with extreme macrocytosis (120 fl) and a low plasma vitamin B12. The anti-parietal cell antibody should be positive.

Temporal Arteritis causes constant headaches with tenderness over the temples. It can cause irreversible bilateral blindness; it responds quickly to steroids.

Depression is a difficult problem in the elderly. I find it difficult to diagnose, but I'm used to blood tests and X-rays. Treatment, even with modern antidepressants, is unsatisfactory. The pills always need time (weeks) to work.

3.7. THE VERY OBESE

Severe obesity is a common clinical problem. It comes with a wide variety of clinical complications (see Table 3.3 and Figure 3.7). Diabetes is typical but not universal, and it has its own complications. The skin suffers: the folds are permanently damp and can become infected. The joints, especially hips and knees, wear out, giving early osteoarthritic problems. The arterial blood pressure can be high. But the major problem for the very obese is the respiratory evil that goes with severe obesity: 'obstructive sleep apnoea' and the related 'obesity hypoventilation syndrome' are the classic complications. In these conditions, overweight patients (typically middle-aged men with thick necks) display abnormal oxygen saturations and blood gases (hypoxia, hypercapnia), with or without disturbances in sleeping patterns at night, morning headaches, daytime somnolence, and signs of right and sometimes left heart failure.

Investigation and assessment of the very obese should include tests of metabolic status, especially blood glucose and arterial blood gases. A sleep study is often useful. An echocardiogram is useful (if technically difficult in this context) to try and assess the pressure in the pulmonary artery.

Treatment for obesity traditionally starts with a diet. Diets certainly work if the patient has the fortitude to stick to them. In spite of all protestations, if the energy intake is significantly less than the expenditure, the patient will lose weight. Look how quickly a patient with a partially obstructed oesophagus sheds the pounds. The problem is in our psychology. Of the alternative measures, only bariatric surgery (some kind of gastric bypass, typically: see Useful Box 3.10) has been shown to work convincingly.

Table 3.3. The Very Obese.

Point	*Comment*
Classic features in a severe case	By definition, a greatly increased body weight, typically over something like 110 or 115 kg, or a body mass index of >40. Limited mobility, joint and skin problems, diabetes, hypertension and sleep apnoea and/or alveolar hypoventilation. Cyanosis, CO_2 retention, sleepiness. Major difficulties in clinical examination, investigation and IV access. It doesn't end here, but the hypoxic/hypercapnic pathology has to be very important.
To look out for	Low oxygen saturation is a key simple test for respiratory problems.
Progression	Complications of diabetes (Section 2.6.1); deteriorating blood gases (Section 3.6); pulmonary hypertension; dyspnoea; heart failure.
Terminal events	Infection; respiratory failure; diabetic vascular complications; malignancy.
Likely causes	If only we understood this one...
Rare but treatable causes	Cushing's, hypothyroidism.
Acute forms	Can present as acute respiratory difficulty.
Tests to be done	Oxygen saturation; blood gases; blood glucose; HbA1C; sleep studies; exclude Cushing's (Section 2.6.3).
Treatment (in addition to that of underlying disease)	You can try suggesting a diet. Thousands have done the same before. Orlistat, inhibitor of lipases, gives your patient steatorrhoea and will not stop carbohydrate absorption. Sibutramine is an amphetamine-like appetite suppressant. But the only real proven successful treatment is bariatric surgery.
Prognosis	Without weight loss, is not good.

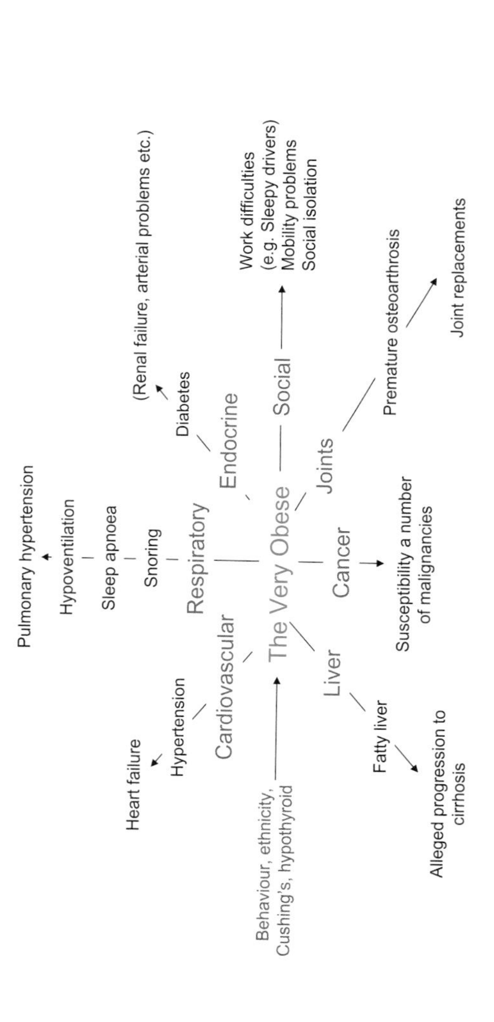

Figure 3.7. Map: The Very Obese. The map summarises the main problems faced by those with substantial body mass index surpluses. Easily the most serious is 'respiratory', but none of the others is trivial either.

Useful Box 3.10. Bariatric Surgery. The word 'bariatric' is derived from a Greek root 'bar' meaning weight. So 'bariatric' means treatment of weight, that is, obesity. The word is nicely euphemistic. As we know, dietary efforts are largely unsuccessful in reducing obesity and at present the pills are not much better. The surgeons have developed useful and effective means of reducing body weight, in which the anatomy of the stomach and small bowel is adjusted to try to provide early satiety and to limit absorption. It is quite major surgery, and obese people are not the easiest to work on, but it really does work as both the statistics and the personal stories of a number of celebrities have demonstrated.

4

Four Lists of Ten

This chapter contains four tables showing what I think are the ten most important emergencies, the ten most common presenting complaints (in hospital), the ten most useful tests and the ten most useful drugs.

This section is as brief as it gets. We have seen virtually everything in these tables before, in one way or another. Like every section of this book, these tables are very far from exhaustive, but they represent the key core areas that I think should be the fundamentals of your knowledge.

In the learning of medicine, emphasis is placed on conditions that are common, life-threatening and curable. Not that many conditions are truly 'curable' (most infections, some cancers possibly), but a great deal of illnesses are least in some way 'treatable'. It is such conditions that are dealt with here.

4.1. THE TEN MOST IMPORTANT EMERGENCIES

The table (Table 4.1) shows what I consider to be ten important emergencies that you need to know about. We are not going to consider the ultimate emergency, 'cardiac arrest'.

'Ventricular tachycardia' is a cardiac arrhythmia one step short of ventricular fibrillation. It is usually a complication of ischaemic heart disease. The ventricles take it upon themselves to beat at a mechanically-inefficient rate of 180–200, at which rate the heart only just sustains an output. It can be treated pharmacologically, but often a DC shock is required to 'reset' the heart.

Raised intracranial pressure is discussed in Section 2.7.2.8.

'Very severe asthma' and 'very severe epilepsy', also known as 'status asthmaticus' and 'status epilepticus' respectively, are conditions in which asthma and epilepsy become life-threatening. The asthmatic lung is very 'tight', so tight that the breath sounds may be almost inaudible; the patient is blue and drowsy with a fast, 'thready' pulse. In severe epilepsy, one fit is closely followed by another, and then another, etc. This anoxic cycle must be interrupted.

Acute pulmonary oedema is a very urgent form of (left) heart failure (Section 2.1). 'Tension' pneumothorax occurs when air can get out of the lung into the pleural cavity but not back again, so that the air builds up in the pleural cavity, taking up more and more space, and compressing both of the lungs and the heart. The key signs are absence of breath sounds on the affected side (which must be resonant to percussion), and deviation of the trachea to the opposite side.

Diabetic ketoacidosis is the metabolic acidosis that occurs in the absence of insulin. A hyperventilating, acidotic patient; ketones in the urine. Temporal arteritis is a 'large vessel' vasculitis in older people that goes for the head and neck. It can affect the central retinal arteries, giving sudden irreversible blindness. It responds quickly to steroids.

Table 4.1. The Ten Most Important Emergencies.

	State	*Clinical*	*Essential Tests*	*Action*
1	Ventricular tachycardia	Rapid, 'thready', regular pulse. Hypotensive.	ECG.	DC shock. Amiodarone. $MgSO_4$.
2	Raised intracranial pressure	Nauseated, vomiting, drowsy, dilated pupils, papilloedema, IIIrd, VIth palsies.	CT head.	Dexamethasone, sometimes surgery if needs be.
3	Very severe asthma	Collapsed, blue, dyspnoeic, widespread polyphonic rhonchi, silent chest.	CXR, gases, try to record peak flow.	O_2, nebulisers, steroids, ventilate.
4	Very severe epilepsy	Recurrent fits.	Blood glucose, U&E, drug levels if relevant.	Diazepam; often paralyse and ventilate.
5	Acute pulmonary oedema	Cold, sweaty, very dyspnoeic. Pink, frothy sputum. Masses of medium crackles in all lung fields.	CXR. ECG.	O_2, morphine, diuretics, IV GTN.
6	GI bleed	Haematemesis, melaena, low BP, postural fall, tachycardia.	Endoscope. PTT.	Transfuse, banding if varices are the cause, surgery.
7	Tension pneumothorax	Blue, collapsed, absent breath sounds on one side. Trachea deviated to opposite side.	CXR (if there is time).	Chest drain.
8	Diabetic ketoacidosis	Hyperventilating, dry, history of thirst and polyuria, ±abdo pain.	Gases, blood glucose, urinalysis (shows ketones).	Insulin, fluids, ±potassium.
9	Spinal cord compression	Neurology with 'level' (Section 2.7.2.6).	MRI cord.	Surgery if needs be.
10	Temporal arteritis	Headache, tender temporals, visual disturbance.	ESR.	Steroids.

4.2. THE TEN MOST COMMON PRESENTING COMPLAINTS

This section could be a textbook in itself, but here goes, 'diagnostic medicine' slashed to the bone. The problems are summarised in Table 4.2.

'Breathlessness' is a very common symptom, and is usually due to lung or cardiac problems. Key diagnoses in these two systems are: exacerbation of COPD, pulmonary embolus, pneumothorax, pleural effusion, 'fibrotic' lung disease, pulmonary oedema. Non-cardiopulmonary causes include very severe anaemia and metabolic acidosis.

Headache is very common. The three big ones are raised intracranial pressure, meningitis and subarachnoid haemorrhage. Non-lethal but troublesome causes include migraine, trigeminal neuralgia, cluster headache and tension headache.

Abdominal pain has a thousand causes. The intestine can ulcerate, block, inflame or perforate. The pancreas can become inflamed. Stones can block bile duct or ureters. Ovaries and uterus can cause grief too. The aorta can dilate up. Vomiting blood is simpler: gastric or duodenal ulceration, or varices.

Chest pain is often caused by ischaemic heart disease, but the oesophagus, trachea, pleural and pericardial membranes can cause pain. The thoracic aorta can stretch or rip.

Fatigue: the hardest. Can be endocrine, renal, rheumatological, neurological or haematological. Or cardiac.

The unconscious patient: has to have something neurological. Raised intracranial pressure is very serious, but rare. Poisoning is a common cause.

Fever: check the CRP (although it can be normal in the first day or two of serious infection). Check all the systems including the heart valves.

Jaundice is typically caused by disease in the liver or by obstruction to the biliary system, but don't forget about haemolytic anaemia (which is 'pre-hepatic' jaundice).

Table 4.2. Ten Most Common Presenting Complaints.

	Complaint	*Main Differential*	*Tests*	*Don't Miss*
1	Breathlessness	Heart or lung problems. Asthma (wheeze); pulmonary oedema (crackles+++); PE (little to find, usually); pneumothorax (absent breath sounds on the affected side).	CXR, gases, CTPA.	Tension pneumothorax.
2	Headache	Meningitis (fever, meningism), SAH (sudden onset, meningism), raised ICP, migraine, tension headache, temporal arteritis.	CT, LP, ESR.	Raised ICP, temporal arteritis.
3	Abdominal pain	Abdo sepsis, GI perforation, obstruction, ischaemia, pancreatitis, aneurysm, biliary and renal colics.	CT abdo, amylase. WBC, CRP.	Perforation.
4	Vomiting blood	Peptic ulcer, bleeding varices.	Endoscope, PTT.	Varices.
5	Chest pain	Angina, pulmonary embolus, pleurisy, aneurysm. oesophagitis, pericarditis.	CXR, ECG, CTPA.	Aneurysm. MI.
6	Fatigue	Endocrine, renal, inflammatory, haematological, psychological.	FBC, U&E, endocrine tests.	Addison's.
7	Unconscious	Drugs (opiates, benzos), raised ICP, stroke, SAH, hypoglycaemia.	CT head, blood sugar.	Hypoglycaemia.
8	Collapsed and re-awoke	Arrhythmia, seizure, faint.	24-hr ECG, CT head, EEG.	
9	Fever	Infection (any system!), lymphoma.	Cultures, FBC, CRP, many scans, echo.	Septic shock.
10	Jaundice	Haemolysis (high bilirubin, ALT, alk phos normal), hepatocellular liver disease (increased ALT), biliary obstruction (increased alk phos).	LFTs, FBC, US liver, CT liver.	Surgically remediable obstruction.

4.3. THE TEN MOST USEFUL TESTS

This is a bit of a cheat because many of the tests here are multi-dimensional. For instance a 'blood count' gives you 7 independent pieces of information (Hb, red cell count. MCV, platelet count, neutrophil, lymphocyte and eosinophil counts.)

We are not including urinalysis here, considering it to be part of physical examination. We certainly cannot do without biopsies and histological examination but they are specialised tests based on many further investigations.

I always like a good blood count. Sick patients are very often anaemic. The size of the red cells tells you about iron, thalassaemias, B_{12}, folate and the patient's alcohol intake. The white count (with differential) is a vital investigation in infection. Platelets tell you about bleeding.

You cannot know about the kidneys (Section 2.5) without the U&E. Sodiums and potassiums are important for body fluids and for the stability of excitable cells.

The liver tests are crucial to sorting out the jaundiced patient. The albumin drops when hepatic synthetic function is poor, or in 'inflammation', or if proteins are being lost through leaky 'nephrotic' glomeruli.

The CRP is a tremendously useful measure of inflammation in all its forms; the chest X-ray is a vital step in the diagnosis of breathlessness; the ECG is vital for sorting out cardiac rhythm disturbances, for diagnosing cardiac ischaemia in all its forms, and pericarditis; the CT head is extremely useful for the assessment of an unconscious patient; the ultrasound of the abdo can show you stones, tumours, collections of pus. It could be argued that a CT would be even better here. Bacterial culture is absolutely invaluable if you can get it.

Lastly, lumbar puncture is key to the diagnosis of meningitis, subarachnoid haemorrhage, multiple sclerosis, viral infections, and idiopathic raised intracranial pressure.

Table 4.3. The Ten Most Useful Tests in Medicine.

	Test	*What it Tells You*
1	FBC	Whether patient is anaemic or not. Size of the red cells (alcohol, iron, B_{12}, folate). White count (infection); platelet count (bleeding).
2	U&E	How the kidneys are working (no other way of knowing this). Sodium and potassium status, relevant to hydration and function of excitable tissues.
3	LFTs	What the liver is like. The albumin level reflects not only liver function but also infection, inflammation, renal protein loss and malnutrition.
4	CRP	Inflammation in all its forms: autoimmune, infective, other. Huge 'dynamic range', from 0–500. Extremely useful 'broad-spectrum' test for diagnosis and for monitoring progress.
5	CXR	Lung parenchyma (oedema, infection, fibrosis, tumour). Pleura (effusion, tumour). Heart size and contour. Pneumothorax. Ribs. Clavicles. Mediastinum: nodes, tumour.
6	ECG	Cardiac rhythm. ST segments and T waves (ischaemia, pericarditis). Myocarditis. Left and right-sided hypertrophies.
7	CT head	Space occupying lesion(s); bleeds; skull fracture; size of ventricles; displacement of midline; oedema in tumour and stroke.
8	US abdo	Collections of pus; biliary or renal obstruction; biliary or renal stones; tumours.
9	Bacterial culture	Bacteriological diagnosis, from pus, sputum, blood, CSF, urine, ascitic, pleural or even pericardial fluid. Identity of bug and antibiotic sensitivity: crucial data.
10	Lumbar puncture	Pressure; biochemistry; protein; glucose; presence or absence of blood; 'oligoclonal bands' in MS; cells: neutrophils, lymphocytes, other e.g. tumour; bacteriology: Gram postive or negative bacteria, TB, fungi; culture: bacteria; PCR: viruses.

4.4. THE TEN MOST USEFUL DRUGS

The pharmaceutical armoury is now a very big one. The World Health Organization 'List of Essential Medicines' runs to 37 pages and about 330 drugs, but I think that if I was allowed only ten these are the ones I would want at UCH. See Table 4.4. To make this reasonable I am confining myself to drugs that can be prescribed by the docs on a general ward. I am excluding specialist treatments such as chemotherapy for cancer, immunosuppression after transplant, sophisticated AIDS treatment, anaesthetics, topical antiseptics, IV fluids, oxygen, blood transfusion. Apart from insulin I am avoiding endocrine replacement.

In addition to prescribed drugs you must have IV saline, but it's not on this list because it is not a 'drug'. Half of the patients in the hospital get it, for fluid replacement after vomiting, diarrhoea, excessive diuretics, haemorrhage, in sepsis: it goes on and on.

Table 4.4. The Ten Most Useful Drugs in Medicine.

	Class	*Drug*	*Utility*
1	Antibiotic	Amoxicillin + clavulanic acid	Best all-round antibiotic.
2	Anticoagulant	Heparin	Treatment and prophylaxis of thrombotic conditions.
3	Diuretic	Furosemide	Cardiac failure, hypertension, oedematous states.
4	Analgesic	Morphine	Addictive, but a highly effective analgesic. Very useful in pulmonary oedema. Causes vomiting.
5	Steroid	Prednisolone	Suppression of pathological inflammation.
6	Diabetic	Insulin	Specific to one disease, but diabetes is a very common one.
7	Bronchodilator	Salbutamol	Asthma is also very common.
8	Anti-psychotic	Haloperidol	Control of delirium, hallucination, psychosis.
9	Anti-convulsant	Lorazepam	Control of seizures.
10	Anti-arrhythmic	Amiodarone	Useful antiarrhythmic (supraventricular and ventricular tachycardias, atrial fibrillation) in spite of its thyroid and lung side effects (which are associated with long-term use).

Abbreviations

Here are definitions of abbreviations used in this book. There is a glossary of clinical terms at the end of the book.

Abbreviation	Meaning
ABG	Arterial blood gases
ACE	Angiotensin converting enzyme
ACEI	ACE inhibitor
ACS	Acute coronary syndrome
ACTH	Adrenocorticotrophic hormone
ADH	Anti-diuretic hormone
AF	Atrial fibrillation
AHA	American Heart Association
AIDS	Acquired immunodeficiency syndrome
Aldo	Aldosterone
ALT	Alanine transaminase
ARDS	Acute respiratory distress syndrome
AP	Alkaline phosphatase
BNP	Brain natriuretic peptide
BP	Blood pressure
CAD	Coronary artery disease
CMV	Cytomegalovirus
COPD	Chronic obstructive pulmonary disease

Abbreviation	Meaning
CRP	C-reactive protein
CSF	Cerebro-spinal fluid
CT	Computerised tomography
CTPA	Computerised tomography pulmonary angiogram
CVA	Cerebro-vascular accident ('stroke'). Can be thrombotic or haemorrhagic
CVP	Central venous pressure
CXR	Chest X-ray
DKA	Diabetic ketoacidosis
ECG	Electrocardiogram
ESR	Erythrocyte sedimentation rate
F1, F2	Junior doctors in first and second years after graduation
FBC	Full blood count
FSH	Follicle-stimulating hormone
GB	Gall bladder
GFR	Glomerular filtration rate
GH	Growth hormone
GHRH	Growth hormone releasing hormone
GI	Gastro intestinal
HA	Haemolytic anaemia
HbA1C	Haemoglobin A1C (glycosylated)
HONK	Hyperosmolar non-ketotic (type 2 diabetic crisis)
HIV	Human immunodeficiency virus
ICP	Intra-cranial pressure
INR	International normalised ratio (between patient PTT and normal control), for monitoring warfarin therapy
ITP	Immune thrombocytopenic purpura
ITU	Intensive care unit
IVDU	Intravenous drug user
JVP	Jugular venous pressure
KGB	Komitet gosudarstvennoy bezopasnosti

Abbreviation	Meaning
LFT	Liver function tests
LH	Luteinising hormone
LHRH	LH releasing hormone (also known as gonadotrophin releasing hormone, GnRH)
LP	Lumbar puncture
LV	Left ventricle
MCV	Mean (red) cell volume
MI	Myocardial infarction
MODS	Multiple organ dysfunction syndrome
MRA	Magnetic resonance angiogram
MRI	Magnetic resonance imaging
MSU	Mid-stream urine
PEFR	Peak expiratory flow rate
PEG	Percutaneous endoscopic gastrostomy
PET	Positron emission tomography
PTT	Prothrombin time
SLE	Systemic lupus erythematosus
T4	Thyroxine
TB	Tuberculosis
TNF	Tumour necrosis factor
Trop T	Troponin T
TSH	Thyroid stimulating hormone
U&E	Urea and electrolytes
UCH	University College Hospital
UCL	University College London
US	Ultrasound
URTI	Upper respiratory tract infection
UTI	Urinary tract infection
WBC	White blood count

Glossary

It is said that in embarking on clinical medicine you have to add more words to your vocabulary than you do when you learn French. Here are my definitions of words used in this book, that might be new to you. I am assuming that you are familiar with anatomical and biochemical terms.

Term	Meaning
Abscess	Collection of pus walled off by an inflammatory reaction.
Acidosis	When the pH of the arterial blood is abnormally low (<7.35). See 'Bad Blood Gases', Section 2.14.
Acquired	*Not* genetic in nature.
Acute phase response	A collection of abnormal blood results that can go with many major tissue injury situations: severe infection, severe inflammation, tissue injury, major surgery, trauma, pancreatitis... it goes on. High CRP, low albumin, normocytic normochromic anaemia, and a number of other less commonly measured changes.

Term	Meaning
Alveolar hypoventilation	When lungs are inadequately ventilated because of a defect in the structure of the chest, or in muscular or neurological function.
Amaurosis fugax	A fleeting loss of vision (say, 10–60 seconds) caused by a tiny embolus in the central retinal artery or a branch thereof. It is a form of transient cerebral ischaemic attack. Think how such a small embolus causes such a striking symptom.
Amiodarone	Iodine-containing anti-arrhythmic drug, toxic to thyroid and lung.
Anaemia	When the concentration of red cells in the blood is low.
Angina	Unless otherwise qualified, means a dull central pain in the chest which comes on with exercise and goes away when the patient stops exercising.
Aneurysm	A condition in which the structure of the wall of a blood vessel is damaged, usually leading to a widening of the vessel at that point.
Aplastic anaemia	State where bone marrow goes on strike and fails to make its cellular products.
Apoplexy	An old word implying 'sudden clinical deterioration', it is now used solely in the term 'pituitary apoplexy'; an unusual, sudden, infarctive process of the gland.
Acute respiratory distress syndrome (ARDS)	A form of pulmonary oedema based on an inflammatory reaction in pulmonary capillaries. Seen in many major illness situations.

Term	Meaning
Aspiration	1. Often means 'aspiration pneumonia', abnormal entry of pharyngeal fluids into bronchial tree with resulting infection in the lungs. 2. Process in which fluid is sucked out of body space by a tube, e.g. from trachea or pleural cavity.
Asthma	Wheezy, reversible bronchial obstruction, immunologically mediated.
Ataxia	An unsteadiness in movement, especially evident on walking as a staggering gait.
Atrial fibrillation	Common cardiac arrhythmia in which regular sino-atrial node pacing is lost, the atrial cells losing their coherent excitation physiology, resulting in entirely irregular ventricular pacing.
B-cell depletion	Technique for cutting down numbers of B-lymphocytes in the body, using monoclonal antibody against B-cells ('Rituximab').
Bacterial endocarditis	Infection on the heart valves.
Bariatric surgery	Gastro-intestinal surgery aimed at getting the patient to lose weight, normally involving some kind of gastric bypass.
Brain natriuretic peptide (BNP)	Peptide which is in fact made by the heart in spite of the name. Blood levels increase in heart failure.
Bronchiectasis	When the bronchi are abnormally dilated (and therefore subject to infection or bleeding) typically because of past destructive infection such as pertussis (whooping cough) or TB.

Term	Meaning
Bronchitis	A respiratory infection affecting mainly the bronchi, rather than the alveoli (pneumonia) or upper airways (upper respiratory tract infection, URTI).
Bronchopneumonia	A bacterial infection of the lung, including the alveoli, involving disparate patches in different lobes, showing up as 'patchy consolidation' on a chest X-ray. Easily the commonest kind of pneumonia.
Bronchoscopy	Examination of the bronchial tree using a flexible or rigid telescope passed down through the larynx.
Bruit	A skooshing sound heard through the stethoscope, over an artery (carotid, subclavian, renal, femoral are all big enough), and caused by turbulent flow in a narrowed artery.
Candidiasis	Infection with the yeast *Candida albicans.*
Cardiogenic shock	In which the blood pressure cannot be sustained because the heart muscle is too weak to generate the pressure. Term is usually used in context of major myocardial infarction.
Cardiomyopathy	State in which the heart muscle does not pump effectively for whatever reason, usually associated with a 'low ejection fraction' on echo.

Term	Meaning
Central pontine myelinolysis (CPM)	A condition in which the pons, or part of it, is to an extent 'demyelinated' (what it says on the tin, the myelin is lost). Most 'demyelination' is autoimmune in origin but in this case it is due to sudden variation in metabolic state, classically low plasma sodium being returned to normal rapidly (so go carefully with those fluids!).
Cerebrovascular accident	A 'stroke'. A sudden neurological problem caused by either thrombosis (commoner) or haemorrhage within the substance of the brain.
Clonus	A repetitive jerking movement elicited by exerting sudden force to stretch a muscle. Seen at the ankle (stretching of gastrocnemius) and the knee (quadriceps). Goes with increased deep tendon reflexes, and typically reflects a severe upper motor neurone problem.
Coagulopathy	When the clotting system is not working and the patient is bleeding because of that. Happens in severe sepsis, amongst other situations.
Chemotherapy	Treatment for cancer aimed at killing rapidly-dividing cells. Kills cancer cells but also some natural cells, especially bone marrow ('bone marrow failure', 'immunosuppression', 'neutropenia') and possibly gut epithelium.

Term	Meaning
(Intermittent) claudication	Vascular condition in which patient suffers pain in muscles of leg (calf, other) when he or she exercises, relieved by rest. Also, 'jaw claudication', which occurs in temporal arteritis, an inflammatory arteritis which affects only the head and neck.
Cognitive	To do with thought and thinking processes.
Comorbidity	The other (usually chronic) conditions from which the patient suffers, which delay recovery from the main illness. Might commonly be diabetes, COPD, ischaemic heart disease, renal or hepatic failure, cancer.
Computerised tomography (CT)	An X-ray technique in which images are obtained from a scanner that circles the body. A computer takes thousands of images and stitches them together into a series of 'cuts' that give remarkable views of the internal anatomy.
Confusion	State of disturbed cognitive function, typically assessed as difficulty with orientation in time, person and place.
Coning	When raised intracranial pressure forces the brain stem down into the foramen magnum, compressing the medulla and inhibiting the respiration control centre.
Contralateral	On the opposite side.

Term	Meaning
Creatine kinase (CK)	Enzyme that metabolises creatine (which is not the same as 'creatinine', please note). The enzyme is released into the blood when muscle cells lyse. High after myocardial infarction and after damage to voluntary muscle, eg rugby.
Creatinine	Waste product of the breakdown of muscle cells. Excreted by the kidney. A rising plasma creatinine is the best measure of renal function in the chronic situation (urine output is the key measure in the acute situation).
Crohn's disease	An inflammatory disease of the intestinal tract, which can affect in patches any part of the GI tract in patches from mouth to anus. The inflammation is granulomatous. The wall of the bowel becomes thickened and can obstruct; loops of bowel can stick together, and fistulae can form between loops of bowel and bowel and bladder. Although 'inflammatory' it is not 'autoimmune'. See Useful Box 2.3.2.
Cryptococcosis	Infection with *Cryptococcus neoformans*. Can include, in its complete form, meningitis, pneumonia and skin rash. Seen in AIDS. See Useful Box 2.10.1.
Cyanosis	A blueness of the body parts, when the amount of deoxygenated blood is greater than 5g/dl. Can be 'peripheral' or 'central'. 'Peripheral' means fingers and toes, and can occur simply by virtue of sluggish flow in a cold limb in a healthy person. 'Central' means in the tongue and lips, and does mean arterial desaturation, which is bad.

Term	Meaning
Cystic fibrosis	Autosomal recessive disease predominantly of lungs, skin and pancreas. Abnormal sodium chloride content of secretions. Defective lung defence against infection.
Debility	When a patient is noticeably weakened by some kind of disease, such that movements are slow, the cough is feeble, eating is difficult, and much help is required for activities of daily living. Patient is liable to infection in chest, urinary tract and skin.
Deep tendon reflexes	Those reflexes which are elicited with a hammer: biceps, triceps, supinator, knee, ankle, jaw. To be distinguished from 'superficial' reflexes (plantar, abdominal).
Delirium tremens	The 'organic psychosis' that can develop in ethanol-addicted patients about 36 hours after cessation of intake. Severe anxiety, sweating, tremor, frightening visual hallucinations, confusion, berserkness.
Delusions	Faulty beliefs. Not the same as 'hallucinations' which are visions or sounds (usually voices) which are seen or heard, but are not real.
Dementia	When cognitive function (in all its forms) is seriously impaired.
Demyelination	Pathological condition in which myelin is lost from neurones. Usually autoimmune in origin, but not always (see 'central pontine demyelination'). Colloquially, 'demyelination' is taken to mean 'due to multiple sclerosis'.

Term	Meaning
Diabetes	Diabetes mellitus (and not 'insipidus' unless specified).
Dialysis	A technique to support those with renal failure. Blood is taken out of the body via a big cannula, anticoagulated, pumped past a 'dialysis membrane' which allows the passage of small molecules (salts, water, urea, many water-soluble waste products) across itself into a dialysis fluid on the other side of the membrane, then returned to the patient after reversal of anticoagulation.
Disinhibited	A state of mind in which the normal civilised restraints on social behaviour are removed.
Dissection, aortic or carotid	In which because of a rupture in the intimal layer of the vessel (possibly at an atheromatous plaque) blood enters the media compartment, drives through it and creates a 'false lumen' where (usually) it eventually clots.
Diuretics	One of a number of salt+water losing drugs, usually meaning a loop diuretic: furosemide or bumetanide.
Diurnal cortisol	When the blood samples for cortisol are taken at (roughly) 0800 and 2400. The natural rise in the morning and fall in the evening are lost when there is uncontrolled cortisol secretion, as in Cushing's.
Dysarthria	In which the patient has difficulty speaking because of a problem in the mouth or the nerves supplying the muscles of the face and mouth, including of course the tongue.

Term	Meaning
Dyskinesia	In which movements are abnormal in spite of normal power. Can be too little (Parkinson's) or too many (e.g. tics).
Dyspnoea	Difficulty in breathing.
Echocardiogram ('Echo')	Ultrasound examination of beating heart.
Ectopic pregnancy ('An ectopic')	Pregnancy developing outside the uterus, usually in a Fallopian tube, rather than the body of the uterus. The pregnancy recruits a blood supply then ruptures into the peritoneal cavity.
Effusion	An abnormal collection of fluid in a potential space (e.g. joint, pericardial and pleural spaces). Fluid in the peritoneal space is called 'ascites'.
Ejection fraction	That fraction of the left ventricle's volume that is pumped out in a single stroke. Should be about 60%, as measured on an echo.
Electrocardiogram (ECG)	Recording of voltages generated by the synchronous action potentials of the heart during its cycle.
Embolic sepsis	When sepsis travels between two anatomical locations via the blood. E.g. in bacterial endocarditis, the infected valves shower the circulation with bacteria and infected particles, which can lodge and infect the eye, brain, joints and bones.

Term	Meaning
Emphysema	When the normal fine spongy structure of the lung is degraded to a coarse, 'cavitated' texture. It's like taking a fine sponge and poking holes in it with your fingers. Nasty little child that you once used to be.
Encephalitis	Inflammation of the brain. Often viral.
Encephalopathy	When the brain (especially the cognitive elements) are not working, often but not always because of some deleterious process in another system ('hepatic', 'hypertensive').
Endarterectomy	Operative procedure in which a narrowing inside an artery is removed.
Exercise tolerance	Term used to describe a patient's limit of exercise: e.g. 'getting to bathroom', '200 yards', 'half a mile'. (No metric units here please. This is about real people.)
Extradural	Outside the dural membrane, between skull and dura.
Extra-pyramidal	In motor system; to do with the regulatory accessory motor functions mediated by the basal ganglia and cerebellum, rather than the motor cortex.
Fasciculation	After a muscle has lost its lower motor neurone innervation it shows a flickering random contraction of the motor units. Seen best in the tongue, if affected. Often seen in motor neurone disease.
Fibrotic	In which the tissue is laden with abnormal collagen-type fibrotic matter.

Term	Meaning
Fibrosing alveolitis	Chronic acquired autoimmune lung condition in which chronic diffuse inflammatory reaction culminates in scarring with fibrosis.
Fistula	Abnormal connection between two epithelial surfaces.
Flaccid	Of limbs: floppy; loose; lacking tone.
Frusicillin	Colloquial ward term for the therapeutic combination of furosemide and an antibiotic (the patient has wet lungs with patchy shadowing on the CXR. You can't make up your mind whether it is infection or pulmonary oedema).
Functional	1. In heart murmurs, when the valve leaks due to stretching of its mountings rather than damage to the leaflets. 2. In medicine as a whole, when a symptom or sign is of psychological origin.
Fundoscopy	Examination of retinae using an ophthalmoscope.
Gag reflex	Contraction of pharyngeal muscles on stroking of the posterior wall of the pharynx. Tests cranial nerves IX and X. Depends on the context, but absence of gag reflex is sometimes assumed to mean that patient may not be able to protect his or her own airway and therefore be liable to develop aspiration pneumonia.
Gangrene	When a part of the body loses its blood supply and cells die *en masse*. The affected part turns black and smells unpleasant, in part due to growth of anaerobic organisms.

Term	Meaning
Gastroenteritis	Infection of the GI tract caused by viruses or bacteria (or other organisms e.g. amoebae) giving nausea, vomiting diarrhoea, abdo pain and fever; or some combination thereof.
Glasgow coma scale	Simple practical scale for assessment of conscious level, measured by observation of eye movements, verbal responses and motor responses (Useful Box 2.32).
Glove and stocking	Sensory loss of the peripheries of the limbs in the areas covered by the items of clothing named. Caused by a general problem in all peripheral nerves, the longest nerves suffering the most.
Gluconeogenesis	The making of glucose from other biochemicals e.g. amino acids. Mainly happens in the liver.
Goitre	Enlargement of the thyroid.
Gout	Inflammation of a joint, commonly the big toe, caused by occurrence of crystals of sodium urate in the structures of the joint, perceived by the body as foreign objects.
Guillain-Barré	Autoimmune peripheral neuropathy, typically affecting motor nerves, which 'ascends': affects feet first then works its way up. Can involve respiratory muscles, which is serious.
Gynaecomastia	Abnormal development of breast tissue in a male, also serious.
Haemophilia	An inherited clotting disorder most often caused by mutations in the factor VIII gene, which is on the X chromosome, so it is an 'X-linked recessive'.

Term	Meaning
Haemothorax	Blood in the pleural cavity (can coexist with 'pneumothorax', especially in trauma).
Haemolytic anaemia	Anaemia due to premature destruction of red cells in the circulation. Most cases are autoimmune, due to circulating antibodies directed against red cells, or congenital, often due to a fault in one of the globin genes.
Hemianopia	Loss of vision from one half of a visual field. Can be 'homonymous', affecting same area of the field in each eye (usually left or right side, and caused by a lesion posterior to the chiasma), or affecting temporal field in each eye, in which case the lesion is at the chiasma itself.
Hemiplegia	Weakness of upper and lower limbs on one side of the body.
Hepatitis	Inflammation in the liver. Can be viral (hepatitis A, B or C), or chemical (ethanol) or automimmune.
Hepatomegaly	When the liver is perceptibly enlarged on physical examination.
Horner's syndrome	Dysfunction of sympathetic supply to head. Partial ptosis, constricted pupil, loss of sweating on affected side, slightly sunken eye. Eye movements are normal.
Hypercapnia	High pCO_2 in arterial blood (>6.1 kPa).
Hypertension	High blood pressure. Unless qualified (e.g. 'pulmonary' or 'portal') means arterial hypertension. Note also 'intracranial hypertension' which is high pressure in the CSF. All of these 'hypertensions' have entirely different causes, please note.

Term	Meaning
Hypoventilation	When the rate or depth of ventilation is insufficient to maintain normal blood gases.
Hypoxia	When the partial pressure of oxygen in the arterial blood is low (less than about 10 kPa).
Idiopathic	Where the cause is not known. The adjective 'essential' is also used to express this state of ignorance: 'essential hypertension'.
Immunosuppression	Pharmacological treatment aimed at damping down aspects of immune function. Would include glucocorticoids, azathioprine, methotrexate, ciclosporin, tacrolimus, others.
Infarction	When a tissue dies from loss of its blood supply, for whatever reason.
Inflammatory bowel disease	Collective term for Crohn's disease and ulcerative colitis, the two chronic gut diseases in which excessive inflammation is a feature. Note that unlike the rheumatological inflammatory conditions, these are not 'autoimmune'. See Useful Box 2.3.2.
'Inotropic support'	Intravenous treatment with catecholamine-type molecules designed to increase the systolic BP and increase renal perfusion.
Intention tremor	Excessive oscillatory movement of a limb which gets worse when the patient sets out to do a task e.g. point at your own outstretched finger.
International normalised ratio (INR)	See 'prothrombin time'.

Term	Meaning
Interventional radiologist	A fancy form of radiologist who moves from a 'simple' diagnostic role into an active person who seeks to treat pathology on his or her table, e.g. opening up tightened or blocked arteries, or embolising tumours. Tend to be rich.
Ionising radiation	Subatomic particles or electromagnetic beams that are sufficiently strong to make atoms gain or lose electrons; equivalent to the ability to damage biological molecules including DNA. X-rays, like gamma rays (a form of electromagnetic radiation), are 'ionising', while visible light is not. Neither magnetic resonance nor ultrasound involves ionizing radiation but CT and plain X-rays do, obviously.
Ipsilateral	On the same side as.
Ischaemia	A shortage of blood supply.
Ketoacidosis	In which a metabolic acidosis is caused by the 'ketone bodies', namely acetoacetic acid and beta-hydroxybutyric acid. These are the acids in the blood in uncontrolled type one diabetes.
Lead-pipe rigidity	A form of muscle rigidity in which the resistance to your pressure is constant throughout the arc of movement. When joint is flexed or extended to given angle, the limb then stays put. 'Lead-pipe' is an old analogy from plumbing. In modern terms, it might better be likened to Plasticine.

Term	Meaning
Leukaemia	A cancer of the blood in which very large numbers of white cells (neutrophils, 'myeloid leukaemia', lymphocytes, 'lymphocytic leukaemia') are seen in the peripheral blood.
Long tracts	In the brainstem and spinal cord, the name given to the motor and sensory 'tracts' passing up and down past the localized site of the lesion under scrutiny.
Lower motor neurone	Motor neurone passing from cord to muscle. Dysfunction of this causes a floppy, flaccid muscle that wastes (loses bulk) and fasciculates (shows random flickering contractions similar to those that you get around your eye when you are tired).
Lymphoma	A cancerous process in the lymphocytes of the lymphatic system. Forms swellings in the lymphatic tissues.
Malabsorption	State where ingested food is poorly absorbed from the gut and emerges unabsorbed in the faeces. In the case of fat, this presents as 'steatorrhoea'. Can be caused by coeliac disease.
Megaloblastic anaemia	Megaloblasts are large red cell precursors seen in the bone marrow, found in peripheral blood in deficiencies of vitamin B_{12} and folic acid; vitamins that are required for effective cell division.
Melaena	Passage of blood in the stool.

Term	Meaning
Meningeal irritation	When the patient has symptoms and signs suggesting that the meninges are angry. Headache, photophobia, difficulty in flexing the neck, pain on raising the leg with the knee extended (straight-leg raise).
Meningism	Showing symptoms and signs of meningeal irritation.
Meningitis	Inflammation, usually infective, of the meninges. Can be bacterial or viral or other microorganisms. Definitive diagnosis by lumbar puncture.
Metastasis	'Secondary' deposit of malignant tumour at a site distant from the 'primary' tumour. Typically the secondary gets there via the blood or the lymphatics, but not always.
Microcytosis	When the red cells in the blood are unduly small. Seen in iron deficiency and thalassaemias.
Mitotic	At the bedside, colloquially means 'malignant'.
Mitral incompetence	When the mitral valve leaks during systole. Pan-systolic murmur at the apex. Tsssst tsssst tsssst, etc.
Multiple sclerosis	Autoimmune neurological disease in which myelin is attacked in patches throughout the central nervous system.
Myelitis	Inflammation, usually autoimmune, in the spinal cord, usually localized to a level.

Term	Meaning
Myelo-	Prefix derived from Greek meaning 'marrow'. Used for either (i) bone marrow (ii) neutrophil cell line ('myeloid') or (iii) spinal cord ('transverse myelopathy' or 'myelitis'). Also used in 'osteomyelitis', infection of bone.
Myelofibrosis	Condition in which marrow is infiltrated by fibrotic tissue, displacing and shutting down haematopoietic tissue.
(Multiple) myeloma	A malignant process of the marrow in which a clone of plasma cells proliferate, often secreting an antibody, which is of course 'monoclonal'. It is from manipulated myeloma cells that monoclonal antibodies are made.
Myelopathy	= myelitis.
Myocarditis	Inflammation of heart muscle, often viral; can be autoimmune. May or may not be destructive to function of heart muscle.
Myopathy	Where the muscles are not working properly because of a defect in the function of the muscles themselves rather than in the nerves that control them.
Naso-gastric	A wee plastic tube passed down through the nose (it's more comfortable in the long term than going through the mouth), down the oesophagus and into the stomach; used either to aspirate stomach contents up, or feed the patient if natural swallowing is not happening.

Term	Meaning
Neurofibromatosis	Inherited condition of the nervous system in which nerves, usually peripheral, have a tendency to form multiple benign tumours.
Neuropathy	Defect in nerve function, typically 'peripheral', i.e. outside the central nervous system.
Neutropenia	Low neutrophil count ($<2.0 \times 10^9/l$). When the neutrophil count is less than about $0.5 \times 10^9/l$ the patient can run into very severe sepsis problems, known as 'neutropenic sepsis'.
Nystagmus	A jerking movement of the eyes, seen in cerebellar, eighth nerve, and some brainstem problems.
Oncology	1. Study of cancer, all aspects of. 2. Clinical service dealing with cancer patients.
Opiate	One of heroin, morphine, codeine and variants derived from the opium poppy, which usually have these properties: strongly analgesic, respiratory depressant, addictive, euphoriant.
Ophthalmoplegia	A defect in the movement of the eyes, often 'external ophthalmoplegia' meaning a problem with the muscles operating eye movements.
Osteoarthrosis (also known as 'osteoarthritis')	'Wear and tear' in joints. Joint pain, stiffness and swelling which is mainly the result of mechanical wear, rather than immune attack from rheumatoid arthritis-type pathology.

Term	Meaning
Osteomyelitis	Infection of bone, typically with staphylococci or TB
Osteoporosis	Diminution in the protein scaffolding of the bone, reducing the available tissue for calcification, weakening the bone.
Palsy	Old-fashioned word meaning weakness, still preserved in 'Bell's palsy', an idiopathic VIIth nerve weakness, named after Charles Bell, one of the founders of UCH. Also, 'cerebral palsy', the result of anoxia at birth.
Pancreatitis	Inflammation of the pancreas. Unpleasant, painful condition often accompanied by very marked inflammatory response equal to that seen in full-scale septic shock. The gland is a storehouse for all manner of biological weapons. Pancreatitis is the pathological equivalent of a fire in a dynamite factory.
Pancytopenia	Shortage of all cellular elements of the blood: red, white and platelet.
Papilloedema	Swelling of the optic disk, visible through the ophthalmoscope as blurring of the disk perimeter, and redness. The optic nerve is ensheathed in a cylinder of dura containing CSF. High CSF pressure is transmitted along this sheath and the ophthalmoscope allows us to see this swelling with the naked eye.
Paraesthesiae	Pins and needles.

Term	Meaning
Paraneoplastic syndrome	In cancer, when a dysfunction occurs in a location or system entirely distinct from the tumour or its secondary deposits. Can be endocrine (secretion of ADH by small cell lung cancer influencing the kidneys) or neurological (cerebellar or basal ganglia dysfunction).
Paranoia	Just because you're paranoid doesn't mean to say that everyone isn't out to get you.
Paraplegia	Weakness of both legs.
Parenteral nutrition	The supply of nutrition to a patient via a vein rather than the GI tract. Comes in the form of a lipid emulsion.
Parvovirus	Virus that has to infect actively dividing cells for its own replication. The canine form goes for the GI tract. The human form causes a mild rubella-like fever, with the nasty occasional complication of aplastic anaemia.
Past pointing	Physical sign of cerebellar disease related to 'intention tremor'. When you ask the patient the patient to reach out and point to your finger, his or her aim is poor.
PEG feeding	Feeding via a tube that passes into the stomach through the abdominal wall. Tube is in fact inserted from the lumen of the stomach back through the abdominal wall using an endoscope.
Photophobia	Dislike of light. Seen in meningism.
Physical sign	An abnormality that is found on physical examination.

Term	Meaning
'Plantar'	Colloquial term for a 'plantar response', in which the plantar aspect of the foot is stroked while the examiner watches the initial movement of the great toe. Normal = down, or 'flexor'; abnormal, and meaning upper motor neurone lesion is present, is up, or 'extensor'.
Pneumothorax	Air in the pleural cavity. Can be 'spontaneous', or traumatic, or secondary to lung pathology such as tumour or emphsema or infection.
Polyphonic	Of wheezes (rhonchi) in the chest that are all of different pitch; the opposite of 'monophonic', in which there is just one sound, caused by a single obstruction (tumour, foreign body) sitting in the bronchus. 'Polyphonic' implies many, many obstructions, i.e. asthma.
Primary biliary cirrhosis	Autoimmune condition of the liver, in which main attack is on small bile ducts, which gradually obstruct. Auto-antibodies found in the blood, usually 'anti-mitochondrial antibodies'.
Proteopathy (alternatively, proteinopathy)	A disease state caused by abnormal and disruptive accumulation of proteins in cells (usually neurones).
Polyarteritis nodosa	Inflammatory arterial condition, typically affecting larger arteries. Can complicate chronic hepatitis B infection.
Postural hypotension	When the blood pressure falls on standing up. Useful sign of 'volume depletion' within the circulation.

Term	Meaning
Pre-renal renal failure	Meaning that the cause of the renal failure is 'upstream' from the kidneys themselves. Basically, poor perfusion from the cardiovascular system. Renal failure can occur from 'renal' causes, within the kidney (e.g. diabetes), or 'post-renal', meaning obstruction to outflow of urine.
Productive cough	A cough in which sputum is produced. Distinct from a 'dry cough'.
Protein C	A 'circulating anticoagulant', a protein found in the blood that has the effect of slowing down blood clotting.
Proteinuria	Presence of abnormally high amounts of protein in the urine, often arising from damaged, leaky glomeruli.
Prothrombin time	A lab measurement of the extrinsic coagulation pathway. Coagulation is started by addition of tissue factor. Result is usually expressed as the 'INR', the 'international normalised ratio', the ratio between the patient sample time and the parallel normal control.
Pulmonary hypertension	When the resistance to flow in the pulmonary system is high. Clinically, associated with dyspnoea, cyanosis, a loud pulmonary valve heart sound, and signs of strain on the right side of the heart on ECG.
Purpura	Spontaneous bruising, basically, with lesions sized 0.3–1.0 cm; petechiae, <0.3 cm; ecchymoses, >1.0 cm.

Term	Meaning
Pyelonephritis	Infection of the pelvis of the kidney. Usually 'ascending' (coming up from the bladder) and usually bacterial, and usually caused by *E coli*. All these bets are off, however, if the urinary tract is anatomically abnormal.
Pyramidal	To do with the main motor pathway from motor cortex to lower motor neurone, as opposed to 'extra-pyramidal', meaning the accessory 'regulatory' motor pathways, basal ganglia and cerebellum.
Retinopathy	Funkiness in the retina, commonly due to bad blood vessels: leaky and blocked (diabetes, hypertension); but can be viral, as in cytomegalovirus retinopathy in AIDS.
Renal artery stenosis	Tightening of the renal artery. If unilateral can cause hypertension; if bilateral or if there is only one kidney it is a cause of renal failure.
Rhabdomyolysis	Rupture of muscle cells, their contents being released into the circulation. In large quantities these breakdown products are toxic to the renal tubules, and are a cause of 'acute renal failure'. Caused by trauma, hyperpyrexia.
Rheumatic fever	Unpleasant post-streptococcal autoimmune disease affecting joints, heart, brain and skin. Anti-streptolysin antibodies in the blood. Can cause chronic scarring effect on endocardium, affecting valves. The acute disease is not common in UK now, but the heart valve problems are seen.

Term	Meaning
Rheumatoid arthritis	Autoimmune disease of synovial membranes. Youngish adult, more commonly female. Symmetrical, small joint arthritis.
Rheumatoid factor	An autoantibody (directed against the Fc fragment of the IgG molecule) present in many patients with rheumatoid arthritis.
Rigidity	A state of increased muscle tone where the resistance to passive movement is increased.
Sarcoid	Idiopathic disease in which 'granulomatous' inflammation occurs in different parts of the body: mediastinal lymph nodes, skin, brain, ... everywhere except the adrenal, apparently.
Sensory level	A finding on physical examination in which one is able to define a boundary, below which sensation is in some way abnormal and normal above it. Goes with spinal cord pathology.
Sickle cell disease	Haemolytic anaemia caused by autosomal recessive defect of beta globin in red cells, in which patients are subject to 'crises'. In a crisis, red cells dehydrate ('dry up'), the intracellular Hb precipitates, the red cells form thrombi, infarcting the bone marrow. The heterozygous state (known as 'sickle cell trait') is protective against malaria.

Term	Meaning
Spider telangiectasia	A telangiectasium is a small abnormal blood vessel on the skin. 'Spider telangiectasia' are vessels that occur in the area of drainage of the SVC. Called 'spider' because they have a central root with branches that spread from the centre like the 8-legged non-flying insect of that name. Seen in pregnancy and in chronic liver disease.
Spina bifida	Developmental accident in the formation of the embryonic neural tube.
Steatorrhoea	Too much fat in the stool. Pale, bulky faeces, a finding in 'gut failure'.
Stent	A tube inserted to open up a narrowed anatomical structure e.g. trachea, bile duct, coronary artery.
Steroid	Typically, means 'glucocorticoid' unless qualified by 'mineralo' or 'sex' or 'anabolic'.
Stridor	Harsh, easily audible inspiratory noise due to narrowing of trachea.
Subacute combined degeneration of the cord	A neuropathy caused by B_{12} deficiency. Affects dorsal (vibration, position) and lateral (motor, sensory) columns in the cord.
Subdural	Deep to the dural membrane, between arachnoid and dura.
Supra-tentorial	Colloquial term for 'psychological'.
Symmetrical	Left same as right.

Term	Meaning
Syphilis	Infection with *Treponema pallidum*. Usually caught venereally. Three stages: primary, secondary, tertiary. Look up 'Isaac Asimov syphilis' on Google.
Takayasu's	An inflammatory arteritis that is found in young adult females of far-eastern origin. Also known as 'pulseless disease'.
Tamponade	When a blood vessel or the heart is obstructed or inhibited by fluid pressing from the outside. Commonly, 'pericardial tamponade' when there is fluid in the pericardial sac.
Tardive dyskinesia	'Dyskinesia' = abnormal movements; 'tardive' = continuing to occur after the supposed cause has been removed, the supposed cause typically being anti-psychotic drugs.
Temporal arteritis	Inflammatory condition of arteries of head and neck seen in older people. It is a cause of blindness, and is always sensitive to steroid treatment. One of the emergencies.
Tension pneumothorax	Pneumothorax in which there is valve-like leak in the lung, which allows air to get into the pleural space but not back out. Air accumulates in the pleural space, compressing lungs and heart. Dangerous, and also one of the emergencies.

Term	Meaning
Tetany	When the muscles begin to contract spontaneously, as a result of a metabolic abnormality, one of alkalosis, hypocalcaemia or hypomagnesaemia. When one or more of these ions (which are small in relation to their charge) are in short supply, neurones can spontaneously activate. Associated with spontaneous sensory symptoms in the form of paraesthesiae. (Note: *not* the same as 'tetanus', in which muscles are paralysed in the contracted state by a circulating toxin from an ischaemic wound contaminated with *Clostridium tetani*.)
Thalassaemia	A series of genetic problems affecting the regulation of globin gene expression. Range in severity from mild to very unpleasant. A cause of microcytosis.
Thrombocytopenia	Shortage of platelets in the peripheral blood.
Thrombolytics	Drugs with ability to break up clots. At present, always enzymes given intravenously.
Thyroiditis	Inflammation of the thyroid gland.
Tissue factor	Protein in extravascular space that activates the 'extrinsic pathway' of blood coagulation.
Tuberculosis (TB)	Infection with *Mycobacterium tuberculosis*, a slowly-growing bacterium which has been described as a 'human commensal organism'. In the disease state, can affect any system, but favourite targets are the lungs and cervical lymph nodes.

Term	Meaning
Tremor	A shaking of a limb or the head. Can be 'resting' (only at rest), 'intention' (during a deliberate act). 'Essential tremor' is a common inherited constant fine tremor.
Ulcerative colitis	An 'inflammatory' (but not autoimmune) condition of the colon. Young adults; diarrhoea with blood and mucus.
Upper motor neurone	The motor neurone that connects motor cortex with lower motor neurone, the connection being at the level where the lower motor neurone exits the cord. Lesions in UMNs give a hypertonic, 'spastic' weakness.
Varices	Very distended veins. In the context of liver disease, refers to 'oesophageal varices', dilated veins at the distal end of the oesophagus, carrying blood on a bypass route from the partly-blocked portal system back to the IVC. They tend to rupture and then bleed profusely.
Vasculitis	Inflammatory condition of the walls of blood vessels, which either get blocked or leak as a result.
Vitreous bleeding	Bleeding into the vitreous compartment of the eye, typically from abnormal blood vessels in the retina, growing there because the originals got blocked.
Volume depletion	Useful phrase to describe shortage of blood in the vascular system.

Term	Meaning
Von Willebrand's disease	Inherited bleeding condition due to defect in von Willebrand factor, a plasma protein that is involved in platelet activation. Can be inherited either as an autosomal recessive or dominant.
Weber syndrome	Classic brainstem stroke event, causing ipsilateral IIIrd nerve palsy, contralateral hemiplegia (corticospinal tract passing through: a 'long tract' sign) and contralateral parkinsonism (connections to basal ganglia).
Wernicke's encephalopathy	Due to thiamine deficiency: acute neurological problem caused by problems in upper part of brainstem and connections. Ataxia, ophthalmoplegia, confusion, memory loss. It is to avert this condition that many alcoholics are given IV vitamins on arrival in Casualty.
Wilson's disease	The copper overload disease. Autosomal recessive. Chronic liver disease with liver failure. In the brain, it is mainly cognitive, motor cortex and basal ganglia. Treatable with copper-chelating agents.